Medica

"Hypnosis is one of the most misunderstood of all medical therapies, yet one of the most valuable. In volume 1 of *Medical Hypnotherapy,* Tim Simmerman reveals how this natural, mind-body technique can be used as an integral part of conventional medicine to prevent pain, diminish fear and anxiety, and relieve suffering. This is one of those unusual books that is accessible to laypersons and healthcare professionals alike. It deserves to be read in every medical school in the nation."

Larry Dossey, MD
Author of *The Extraordinary Healing Power of Ordinary Things*

"Volume 1 of *Medical Hypnotherapy* is a fantastic book. It should be 'must reading' for all medical students, interns, residents, and anyone who works in clinical settings. I wish I'd had this information twenty years ago!"

Christiane Northrup, MD
Author of *The Wisdom of Menopause* and *Women's Bodies, Women's Wisdom*

"An excellent resource, which every healthcare practitioner and patient should read. The information contained in this book will truly educate the practitioner and help the practitioner create a healing relationship and environment. I know from experience that medical education informs us but does not educate us in a way that enables us to help the patient and their experience of an illness and its treatment. volume 1 of *Medical Hypnotherapy* does the job with its insights, techniques, and wisdom."

Bernie Siegel, MD
Author of *Love, Medicine & Miracles* and *Help Me to Heal*

"Tim Simmerman had the 'fire in the belly' to help people empower themselves when he first attended classes at my Hypnotism Training Institute of Los Angeles fifteen years ago. He has since created one of America's finest and most comprehensive hypnotherapy training programs and has trained hundreds of hypnotherapists. Tim's new book, *Medical Hypnotherapy* is an excellent 'field guide' for accelerated healing and pain control with hypnosis."

Gil Boyne, CHt
Executive Director,
American Council of Hypnotist Examiners
Author of *Transforming Therapy*

"I have witnessed wonderful clinical results from techniques presented in *Medical Hypnotherapy*. As a dental practitioner, I've seen clients who have experienced previous physical and emotional dental traumas. Tim Simmerman offers methods to effectively promote healing at deeply profound levels. This pioneering work has great application not only to dentistry, but also with all of healthcare."

Michael Davis, DDS
Smiles of Santa Fe

"Volume 1 of *Medical Hypnotherapy* is written in a well organized and easy to understand style that makes it very user-friendly. It is a 'must read' for counselors interested in helping clients who are dealing with medical issues."

Peggy Lesniewicz, Ph.D., LPCC, LSW, CHt

MEDICAL HYPNOTHERAPY
VOLUME ONE

Principles
and
Methods
of Practice

TIM SIMMERMAN

Published by: **Peaceful Planet Press**
               509 Camino de los Marquez, Ste. 1
               Santa Fe, NM 87505
               www.peacefulplanetpress.com

Copyright © 2007 by Tim Simmerman

Editors: Nate Daly (Master Word Smith), Barbara Gordon, James Serendip
Publishing Consultant: Ellen Kleiner
Peer Review Committee: Robert Sapien, MD, CHt, Peggy Lesniewicz, PhD, CHt, Gil Boyne, CHt, Patrick Singleton, NLPP, CHt
Book design and production: Janice St. Marie
Cover design: Tim Simmerman and Janice St. Marie
Model: Theresa Downs
Technique photos: Daniel Barsotti
Tim Simmerman photo: Heather Simmerman

All rights reserved. No part of this book may be reproduced in any form whatsoever without written permission from the publisher, except for brief quotations embodied in literary articles or reviews.

Printed in Canada on 30% postconsumer recycled paper

Publisher's Cataloging-in-Publication Data

Simmerman, Tim.

    Medical hypnotherapy / Tim Simmerman. -- 1st ed. -- Santa Fe, N.M. : Peaceful Planet Press, 2007.

    v. ; cm.

    ISBN-13: 978-0-9791879-0-2
    ISBN-10: 0-9791879-0-7
    Includes bibliographical references and index.
    Contents: v. 1. Principles and methods of practice --

    1. Hypnotism--Therapeutic use--Handbooks, manuals, etc. 2. Autogenic training--Handbooks, manuals, etc. 3. Alternative medicine. 4. Self-help techniques. I. Title.

RC495 .S56 2007   2007920079
615.8/512--dc22   0707

10 9 8 7 6 5 4 3 2 1

Disclaimer

The contents of this book are for educational and self-improvement purposes only, and not intended in any way to be a replacement for the diagnosis or treatment of any psychiatric, psychological or medical ailment. Hypnotherapy is not a medical procedure, nor is it the practice of medicine. The term medical hypnotherapy is used for name recognition purposes only. Persons with an ailment or any kind of physical complaint for that matter, are to see their physician first, for medical treatment and make use of hypnosis and hypnotherapy as an adjunct to medical treatment, second. Because hypnosis and hypnotherapy methods are a series of self-help skills and their effectiveness depends on the client, no guarantee can be made regarding results of their use. Also for this reason, hypnotherapy practitioners typically refer to the people they work with, and/or teach hypnosis to, as clients or co-hypnotists.

Acknowledgements

I acknowledge the peer review committee members: Robert Sapien, MD, FAAP, CHt; Peggy Lesniewicz, PhD, LPCC, LSW, CHt; Gil Boyne, CHt; and Patrick Singleton, NLPP, CHt for their time and valuable feedback. Their expertise helped this book become an even more useful tool for teaching medical hypnotherapy. I thank all my medical professors, hypnotherapy instructors and self-help trainers for their knowledge. To the Hypnotherapy Academy of America staff and agents for positive change, I acknowledge your dedication to those we train in these methods, the real difference you make every day of every semester and to your collective contribution to the field of hypnotherapy.

*I dedicate this book to you, the reader.
By choosing hypnotherapy to help others use
their inner resources for self-healing,
you become an agent for positive change in the world.*

CONTENTS

Foreword   11
Robert E. Sapien, MD, FAAP, CHt

Introduction   15

Chapter 1
Fundamentals of Therapeutic Hypnosis   17

Chapter 2
Increasing Responsiveness to Hypnotic Techniques   31

Chapter 3
Methods to Induce Hypnosis   51

Chapter 4
Deepening and Testing Techniques   75

Chapter 5
Using the Right Script to Accelerate Healing   95

Chapter 6
Speaking Subconscious: Designing Therapeutic Suggestions and Healing Imagery   107

Chapter 7
Important Influences on Pain Erasure and Accelerated Healing   127

Chapter 8
Overcoming the Roadblocks to Healing and Pain Relief   135

Chapter 9
Dim It Down **147**

Chapter 10
Dilution Is the Solution **155**

Chapter 11
Laying-On of Hands **163**

Chapter 12
Amelioration by Dissociation **179**

Chapter 13
Supporting the Immune System and Self-Hypnosis
  Training Methods **187**

Chapter 14
An Introduction to Noetigenesis and Developing
  Your Healing Presence **203**

Appendix – Scripts
A – Two-Finger Eye Closure **211**

B – Flashlight **215**

C – Ideomotor / Pendulum **219**

D – Two-Finger Eye Closure
  with Disappearing Numbers **227**

E – Hand Press **235**

F – Sequential Imagery **241**

G – Elman's Magic Spot (Pediatric)
  Sapien/Simmerman Modified Version **245**

Bibliography **247**
Index **251**

Foreword

University of New Mexico Pediatric Emergency Department, September 2005
An eighteen-year-old female presents with sudden onset of abdominal pain. On physical examination, she is distressed, and her abdomen is diffusely tender. Her physician recommends blood tests and intravenous access to administer pain medications. She is crying and refuses, saying, "I don't like needles!" After trying to convince her, medical and nursing staff frustration rises.

This situation could be more healing for the patient and less frustrating for the staff caring for her, by following the types of procedures discussed in this book, resulting in the following scenario:

> She is offered relaxation by a certified hypnotherapist who also happens to be her attending physician. With a simple flashlight induction, she easily enters a calm, hypnotic state. The nursing staff prepares to draw her blood and her hypnotherapist/physician suggests that she is calm and that she begins a mental journey. It is also suggested that she feels the nurses working on her arm, but it "just doesn't bother her." The blood draw is unsuccessful. She brings herself out of hypnosis disappointed and anxious. Her hypnotherapist/physician questions her about her angst. She describes a scene as a child where she witnessed her cousin self-injecting heroin. The cousin ultimately lost his arm. The attending physician tells her

that since she was so good at hypnosis they could do a process in which she neutralizes emotions about the childhood scene. She is willing, and the feelings are neutralized.

The second attempt to draw blood is not only successful, but she actually does not realize it had even occurred. She receives intravenous medication for comfort. While she is waiting for the laboratory results, she calls her attending physician/hypnotherapist into the room, and says, "I am a professional photographer. When I travel, will all emergency rooms have someone to help me do that? What was that? What do I need to ask for next time?"

This is just one of many tremendously satisfying situations in which I have used the body-mind connection acutely with hypnosis and hypnotherapy in the Emergency Department. As a clinician I have witnessed the calming, yet powerful effects of hypnosis on my patients, their families and staff—it is a gift. As a certified hypnotherapist, I also use hypnotherapy to help many clients outside of the clinical setting to achieve personal healing mentally, spiritually, and even physically.

As a researcher and educator, with the aid of Tim Simmerman, I have trained physicians and emergency medical technicians (EMTs) in healing language and simple hypnosis using the techniques and tools outlined in *Principles and Methods of Practice,* volume 1 of *Medical Hypnotherapy.* This book serves as a textbook for our trainings both for healthcare providers and hypnotherapists. Mr. Simmerman is a talented and natural teacher. In this book he shows how techniques he teaches in the classroom can be applied in medical situations from the emergency scene, the examination room, the operating room, and on to subsequent healing.

Principles and Methods of Practice, volume 1 of *Medical Hypnotherapy* is a practical straightforward guide for three major audiences: health care providers of all levels including EMTs, physical therapists, nurses, midlevel providers and physicians wishing to provide their patients with comprehensive care; counselors and hypnotherapists seeking to expand their skills in applying hypnotherapy to health care; and individuals interested in the effective use of the mind in healing.

The simple, concise layout provides the reader with a step-by-step approach to engage an aspect of human nature not often appreciated and vastly underutilized—the mind. Because the mind has been and always will be a powerful resource, clinical hypnotherapy supercedes fads or trends in medicine; it should be a mainstay of modern healthcare. Every patient and those who care for them, families and healthcare providers, could benefit from clinical hypnotherapy. I believe the book's impact on modern healthcare will be invaluable and soon realized.

—Robert E. Sapien, MD FAAP, CHt
Chief of Pediatric Emergency Medicine Division
and Associate Professor
University Hospital, Albuquerque, New Mexico
Associate Instructor
Hypnotherapy Academy of America

Introduction

With only minutes of instruction in specific hypnosis methods, healthcare providers of all levels can use hypnotherapy to help the overwhelming majority of sick or injured people reduce or even eliminate their pain and suffering, heal faster, and avoid potential complications from medical procedures. Also with the use of hypnosis, people respond better to medical treatments and are more likely and able to participate in their own recovery. Scientific data about medical hypnosis from various reputable researchers and institutions, such as the Mayo Clinic and the National Institutes of Health, have provided abundant evidence of the value of integrating hypnotherapy into our approach to wellness.

The hypnotherapy methods presented in this book are all natural, gathered by observing people who naturally control pain and think and act in ways that lead to faster healing and illness prevention. From this information, systems and strategies have been created that everyone can learn and benefit from.

Principles and Methods of Practice, volume 1 of *Medical Hypnotherapy*, has been organized according to the way I train people for hypnotherapy certification at the Hypnotherapy Academy of America. The material, however, has been condensed since it would not be possible to include every aspect of the certification program, which entails hundreds of hours of instruction and guided practice. Still, the book will lead you clearly and succinctly to an understanding of the fundamentals of medical hypnotherapy and how to make use of its methods to benefit you and your clients or patients. I can already envision you making use of the principles found within to bring about more health and wellness. I also see the people you help thanking you for investing your time and energy in learning these valuable skills.

CHAPTER

Fundamentals of Therapeutic Hypnosis

To understand therapeutic hypnosis is to comprehend the very nature of human miracles. While conventional medicine saves lives daily, by using hypnotherapy even more can be done to relieve suffering, speed recovery from injury, regain health from disease, and prevent illness. Medical treatments can eradicate most infectious bacteria, excise tumors, and reduce fractures, but they cannot eliminate unhealthy attitudes that hinder healing, reduce immunosuppressive stress, or tell a fetus to turn head-down in the thirty-seventh week of gestation—such results can only be achieved by the mind of the client. The great gift of therapeutic hypnosis is that it mobilizes inner resources latent in every person to aid in healing. This book explains in detail how these resources are harnessed and utilized through hypnosis.

The Definition of Hypnosis

Hypnosis is a natural yet altered state of mind, in which the critical faculty is relaxed and selective thinking is established. In this context, the word *natural* means that everyone has the capacity to enter into the altered state of awareness we refer to as hypnosis.

Everyone enters altered states naturally in the course of their everyday activities. Any time your awareness wanders away from the analytical, reasoning mind you are entering what is called an *altered state*. For example, when you take a nap your brain-wave activity changes from beta to alpha wave function, at which point you are in an altered state. As you continue to nap, your brain shifts to theta and delta wave activity, a change that also takes place in hypnosis.

Daydreaming is another example of a naturally occurring altered state. While daydreaming, you can become so involved in the imaginary situation and the feelings it generates that your body begins to react as if the events were real, causing you to enter into a light hypnotic state, and then particular physiological changes follow. For instance, I know if I daydream about river rafting down the Taos Box on the Rio Grande, my heart beats faster and my muscles tense up as if to hold me safely in the boat while navigating a Class IV rapid. Intensely focused attention naturally alters our state of consciousness, as well. For example, when you are so strongly focused on a project that noises like a telephone ringing or human voices do not distract you, it is likely you are in a light hypnotic trance. Similarly, you may slip into an altered state of consciousness while driving home from a strenuous day at work. Deep in thought about the day's events, you drive on autopilot and suddenly pull into your driveway feeling like only minutes have passed, even though the drive home was actually over half-an-hour.

An altered state, including a hypnotic trance, can even be activated by intense emotion. The resulting shift in consciousness would explain, for example, how a woman who has been traumatized in a traffic accident can, with seeming superhuman strength, lift up the end of her car to rescue her child trapped underneath.

The *critical faculty*, the second component in the definition of hypnosis, begins developing around age seven and serves as gatekeeper to the subconscious mind. It compares new information or stimuli with ideas and beliefs already held in the subconscious. It then determines if the current situation matches a pattern that already has a programmed response in the subconscious mind, or if it calls for further analysis by the conscious mind. During hypnosis, relaxation of the critical faculty facilitates communication between conscious and subconscious levels of awareness. This communication allows beneficial suggestions such as, "Your immune system works more powerfully today than ever before, Mr. Jones," to be accepted and acted upon without having to pass through the processing of the conscious mind.

Finally, *selective thinking* is an increased mental involvement with ideas being presented. Selective thinking is different from concentration. Concentration is a more strenuous focus upon an idea, while selective thinking tends to be effortless participation in an idea. Paradoxically, selective thinking is both a way into, and an effect of, being in hypnosis. This is because the increased ability to hold an exclusive focus makes it easier to communicate accurately and effectively with the subconscious mind. Understanding that the altered state (hypnosis) is naturally occurring, and knowing the characteristics of the critical faculty and the action of selective thinking, are crucial to your successfully inducing hypnosis. They are expanded on later in this chapter, as well as in Chapters Two through Four, which show you how to prepare the client for hypnosis, then how to induce, deepen and test the hypnotic state.

Characteristics of the Hypnotic State

Gil Boyne, a twentieth-century pioneer in hypnotherapy and operator of the first school of hypnotism licensed by a board of education, ascribes three identifying characteristics to the hypnotic state:

- an emotionalized desire to fulfill suggested behavior
- a heightened responsiveness to instruction
- an extraordinary quality of mental, emotional, and physical relaxation.

The subconscious acceptance of therapeutic suggestion creates the first characteristic of the hypnotic state, an *emotionalized desire to fulfill suggested behavior*. Therapeutic suggestions are ideas put forth to be accepted and acted upon by the subconscious mind. Suggestions can encourage either an experience, such as feeling safe and calm in a particular situation, or a behavior, like making healthier food choices. Suppose, for example, a client needs a magnetic resonance imaging (MRI) scan, but, having been claustrophobic in similar situations before, is afraid to have the study done. While he may rationally understand the need for the scan, part of him just does not want to go through with it. This is the perfect time for the use of hypnosis and therapeutic suggestion. With a five- or six-minute medical hypnotherapy session, ideas about feeling safe and comfortably remaining still during the MRI will be accepted and acted on by the patient's subconscious mind. This will help him "feel" like going through with the scan and therefore he will do so far more easily. How this occurs is covered later in this chapter with the explanation of the qualities of the subconscious mind.

The *heightened responsiveness* to instruction, also characteristic of the hypnotic state, means that when new or complex behavior (especially when it seems beyond conscious control) is suggested, the subconscious mind accepts the instruction and the individual acts accordingly. For example, clients in the hypnotic state can be instructed to direct the immune system to put more immunoglobulin into the saliva, which the responsive subconscious mind will then do.

The hypnotic state's third identifying characteristic, an *extraordinary quality of mental, emotional, and physical relaxation,* has seemingly endless applications in medicine. Through hypnosis, a client can be shown in seconds how to stop the flow of anxious thoughts, for example, during a medical emergency. When the mind becomes serene, the emotions calm down and the body follows suit. The client's heart rate and respiration are normalized and medical practitioners can continue with procedures and treatments.

How Hypnosis Affects the Autonomic Nervous System

The following diagram shows how medical hypnotherapy, when used properly, influences the autonomic nervous system.

The Power Perception Has on the Body

The way we perceive a situation influences our subconscious response to it. At the same time, subconscious associations and programming have already influenced our perception of the situation. This paradox, called a tangled hierarchy, is a bit like the old chicken-or-the-egg dilemma. Because the subconscious mind functions as an association-making mechanism, our perception of any given situation is always influenced to some degree by how our subconscious mind associates what is happening in the present with what we have experienced in the past. But even these past perceptions were influenced by subconscious associations already present, so the very associations that limit our present perception

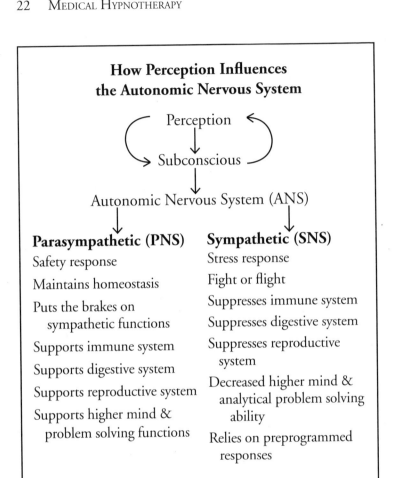

FIGURE 1–1

are themselves limited to some degree. To illustrate this dynamic relationship, Figure 1–1 shows an arrow leading from perception to the subconscious mind and another from the subconscious mind back to perception.

The diagram also depicts the flow of information from the subconscious mind to the autonomic nervous system. Research by Dr. R. Jana at the University of India has shown that every function of the autonomic nervous system can be influenced by the subconscious mind. This implies that every organ, gland, and system of the body is affected by subconscious direction.

The autonomic nervous system branches into two parts: the sympathetic nervous system (SNS) and the parasympathetic nervous system (PNS). Each system becomes activated by a different set of perceptions, contributing to a unique array of physiological changes.

The Sympathetic Nervous System

Whenever stress or danger is perceived, the SNS is activated, resulting in what is known as the fight-or-flight response, which causes a cascade of changes to take place in the body. Blood flow is instantly redistributed away from the gut and pelvic organs and toward the heart, lungs, and large muscles. Vasoconstriction (tightening of blood vessels) occurs, shooting blood to the tissues needed to fight or flee from the dangerous or stressful situation. The immune, digestive, and reproductive systems are instantly suppressed so that energy can be diverted to the systems of the body needed for surviving the immediate stressful circumstance.

In addition to all the physiological changes, significant psychological and emotional changes also occur when the SNS is activated. Fear, which says, "Stop! Go the other way," or anger and rage, which say, "Beat the danger back," are often felt when the SNS is active. When an emergency is perceived, these types of preprogrammed subconscious responses take priority over higher-mind analysis, which requires too much time to be of use. In fact, all the fight-or-flight responses of the subconscious mind spring into effect with peak efficiency whether the trigger is *real or imagined.*

Because of its success in activating the SNS to move us away from danger and pain and toward safety and pleasure, the subconscious mind is often referred to as the survival mind. Developed over thousands of years, this mechanism has certainly contributed to the survival of the human species. It was especially useful in the distant past when people were fleeing from saber-toothed tigers or fighting off invading tribes that were attempting to steal food supplies.

In today's more civilized world, where saber-toothed tigers no longer exist and it is unlikely that a neighboring tribe would steal your bologna sandwich, the subconscious mind can cause harmful physiological changes during situations that are perceived as stressful. Imagine, for example, slugging down a cup of coffee and some Danish before jumping in your car and heading off to work. After being stopped by three traffic lights in a row, you realize you're running late. Remembering the admonition in your last work review that tardiness was to be corrected or you would be put on notice, beads of sweat form on your forehead, your heart starts to beat faster, and the Danish you had for breakfast sits like a rock in your stomach because your sympathetic nervous system has suppressed your digestive function. Speeding up the on-ramp to the highway, you notice a huge eighteen-wheeler alongside you barely giving you room to merge while a car behind you, forced to slow down, honks as if to say, "Hey! Who do you think you are? I'll get you for that!" As you remember the road rage shooting featured on the ten o' clock news last Friday, your foot automatically (subconsciously) presses down on the accelerator. Not noticing the red and blue lights flashing behind you in your desperation to get to work on time, you are shaken out of your trance by wailing sirens. Minutes later, not only are you terrified of losing your job, but you are holding a $100 speeding ticket and the documentation your automobile insurance company needs to increase your premium.

Such scenarios are common in modern-day life. The chronic stress resulting from them is a major contributor to America's current health crisis, as substantiated by an article in *Harvard Mental Health Update*, reporting that 80 percent of all doctor's office visits are stress related.

The Parasympathetic Nervous System

When safety is perceived, the SNS is suppressed and the parasympathetic nervous system (PNS) becomes active. This action puts the body back into balanced function, or homeostasis. Blood flow throughout the body is restored to normal, the reproductive system returns to full healthy functioning, and the digestive system resumes its work of breaking down food into the fuel needed to both run the body and empower the immune system to protect and heal it.

Emotionally, activation of the PNS initiates a shift from fear and anger to calmness and joy. The difference is night and day. Intellectually, in the perceived absence of danger or stress, higher-mind analytical thinking and problem solving are allowed full functioning.

Using the power of perception, with its real and imagined triggers, is instrumental in achieving results through medical hypnotherapy. Couple the induction of hypnosis, which interrupts stress signals to the autonomic nervous system, with the programming of therapeutic suggestions to promote natural PNS function and it becomes possible to effectively prevent disease and accelerate healing.

The Simmerman Model of the Triune Mind

Mind is not brain. Think of it this way: mind is the software and brain-body is the hardware. As Max Planck remarked in his Nobel Prize acceptance speech, mind is the matrix of all matter. Mind is the cause, and body is the effect. Current research shows that the body is a reflection of the mind and they intermingle so intimately that it's nearly impossible to distinguish between them.

Whereas the mind is generally said to comprise two aspects, the conscious and subconscious, the Simmerman model of the mind has three distinct aspects, referred to as levels of awareness. Each level of awareness—conscious, subconscious, and superconscious—has distinct capabilities (resources) and serves different functions. (See fold-out page at end of book.)

The Conscious Level of Awareness

The conscious mind is the reasoning mind, capable of both deductive and inductive reasoning. It is also where volition—making a decision—occurs and then willpower is utilized to accomplish its task. When the conscious mind accepts an idea or decides that something is true, the critical faculty sends the information to the subconscious mind, where it is then sorted, cataloged, labeled, and stored. While the conscious mind seems to operate autonomously, conscious attitudes and inclinations are influenced by fixed ideas held at the subconscious level of awareness.

A key element of the conscious mind is the critical faculty—gatekeeper to the subconscious mind. Its function is to compare new information with ideas already held in the subconscious mind. If new information matches with previously accepted information, the critical faculty opens the gate and allows the new data to enter the subconscious mind. If the new information conflicts, the critical faculty kicks it up to the conscious mind for further analysis. In this way, the critical faculty interprets present events through the filter of past programming, which becomes increasingly fixed in the subconscious mind as we grow older.

The Subconscious Level of Awareness

The subconscious mind is the creative intelligence that runs the body. It influences everything from metabolism and blood pressure to how often we blink our eyes and even how quickly we recover from surgical procedures. It also sorts, catalogs, labels, and stores memories of past events and our interpretations of them. The subconscious mind is often referred to as the subjective mind, because we personally interpret the events we experience and store this as memory. Everything perceived by the subconscious mind is seen through the lens of previous programming. This explains why two people can witness the same event, but later give very different accounts of what happened. Memory is a mixture of fact and perception because the subconscious mind does not distinguish between the two. At the subconscious level of awareness we make subjective interpretations of actual events and store this subjective interpretation as memory.

The subconscious mind does not differentiate fact from fantasy. Research has shown that watching an event and vividly imagining it result in similar physiological responses. For instance, if awakened from a nightmare in which you were chased by a gruesome monster and experienced fear, your heart rate will probably be accelerated, your breathing rapid, and your palms sweaty. In this case, the dream imagery activating your SNS caused a real fight-or-flight response even though you were actually safe in bed.

Further, the subconscious mind receives, stores, and generates imagery, which is a form of language for subconscious thought. For instance, when you have a dream, your subconscious mind relays information to you through images as well as sounds and verbal messages. The images are the "word pictures" your subconscious intelligence is using to communicate.

It is crucial for medical practitioners and hypnotherapists alike to understand that words spoken in the vicinity of sick or injured people form word pictures in their subconscious minds and that, depending on their quality, these internal representations can either cause harm or promote healing.

The subconscious mind also uses the language of emotion. This form of communication reflects the quality of ideas active in the subconscious mind. We feel pleasant emotions when positive ideas are subconsciously active, and for that matter, heavy emotions with negative ideas. Have you ever felt an emotion that you tried to consciously will away, but it only became stronger? This occurs because the seat of emotion is the subconscious mind, not the conscious mind. In its capacity as an association-making mechanism, the subconscious mind constantly links present situations with past events that are in some way similar. Then, based on its interpretation of these events, the subconscious mind fires off emotions to communicate to us whether the present situation is good or bad, safe or dangerous, wanted or unwanted.

Understanding the language of the subconscious mind (see Chapters Five and Six) enables you to communicate and direct this powerful resource.

The Superconscious Level of Awareness

The superconscious mind is your great problem-solving resource. Thomas Edison, who reportedly hypnotized himself to solve problems related to his inventions, received answers to his questions from what he called the "Universal Intelligence." Similarly, in the Polynesian Huna tradition of the South Pacific it is taught that we all have a "high-self," a wise and all-knowing part that can give us important knowledge. I call the seat of this awareness the superconscious mind. Other terms, like "infinite intelligence" or "God mind," have also been used to describe this mysterious part of us.

Many attributes of the superconscious mind are important to medical hypnotherapy. The inner guidance or intuitive knowing it provides can be extremely beneficial to the healing process. Case studies report numerous instances in which intuitive knowing guided people to proper treatment for their illness. The hypnotherapist's work is to help clients free themselves from the subconsciously held limiting beliefs that are reflected in self-defeating thoughts and emotions that slow healing and generate pain. With the amending of such counterproductive programming a latent optimism is revealed and the natural qualities of the superconscious, their divine nature, can emerge. The methods, which are covered in later chapters, often involve the practices of forgiveness, encouraging self-love, and extinguishing any notion of being unworthy of grace—thus allowing healing to occur.

When this level of consciousness is reached in a hypnotherapy session, even if only for a few minutes, the hypnotherapist must make use of it as an ally to facilitate the client's breakthrough. It brings light to the dark thoughts held by the mind that are often the ultimate reason for disease. The superconscious illuminates hidden conflicts and reveals solutions. Hypnotherapy helps the client return to a healthy balance of all three aspects of the mind working together.

CHAPTER 2

Increasing Responsiveness to Hypnotic Techniques

While its roots are ancient, medical hypnotherapy is a modern-day science, which makes use of the latest research and techniques to mobilize inner resources for prevention of disease, acceleration of healing, and pain control. Trance has been used for healing throughout history. It is perhaps the oldest form of healing. For thousands of years, shamans, priests and priestesses conducted rituals and ceremonies with their colorful dress, magical potions concocted from secret sources, and mysterious incantations designed to harness the awesome power of the gods to heal. Essentially, they were inducing an altered state and delivering therapeutic suggestions. Through the use of ceremony, the shaman established a link from the conscious and subconscious to the superconscious, which removed the psychological barriers to wellness and freed the body to heal itself. While modern medicine is an extremely effective tool, the client who consciously desires, but subconsciously resists health, still needs the medical hypnotherapist to "cast the spell" of wellness upon them. This removes psycho-emotional impediments to healing by aligning the subconscious and conscious levels of awareness, thereby increasing the client's responsiveness to their physician's prescribed treatment. While the shaman's healing rituals date back to pre-rational civilization, the principles that induced the trance then still operate today.

The Formula For Hypnotic Induction
The formula for hypnotic induction is: Excited Imagination + Expectation + Refocused Attention = Hypnosis (EI + E + RA = H).

This formula, which is an adaptation from both Bernard C. Gindes and Gil Boyne, indicates the three mental states the client must develop in order to achieve hypnosis. All three ingredients are required, and need to be cultivated in the order presented.

Excited imagination is cultivated by stimulating the subconscious mind of the client with the possibilities made available to them by the use of hypnosis and hypnotherapy. Excited imagination is akin to a positive belief. Belief, according to the dictionary, is the acceptance by the mind that something is true or real, and is often underpinned by an emotional or spiritual sense of certainty. Exciting the imagination is the obvious first step in the hypnotic induction because it begins to engage the client in the process mentally and emotionally. You excite the client's imagination by explaining what is possible for them through using their inner resources, and helping them to picture a positive outcome from the hypnosis session. With an excited imagination, the subconscious is already becoming responsive to positive suggestion.

To expect something is to look forward to it confidently. *Expectation* includes eagerness. Eager expectancy flows out of an excited imagination. It's the feeling of looking forward to the hypnotic experience combined with confidence in the operator. You will inspire this confidence in the client by what you say and how you behave. Master hypnotherapists do not ask the client to have confidence in them, they show the client that they can have confidence in them.

Here are two ways to help with building positive expectancy: first, choose your words intentionally. Avoid slang terms, vernacular and lazy speech. Hypnotherapy demands the skillful use of language. Speak intelligently, but not over the client's head. Teach, don't tell. Ask whether the client has ever seen someone be hypnotized or been hypnotized themselves. Then, based on their answers, you can teach about hypnosis from their point of reference.

Second, let your behavior express an easy and calm confidence. Your hand gestures, body posture, facial expressions, the tone and tempo of your speech—all combine to signal ease and confidence. Behave with the intention of being a trustworthy guide, someone who has been there before and can handle whatever comes up. That will help your client to more easily develop strong positive expectancy.

Refocused attention is the formal induction process. Let's look at the sequence of events in the first session with a new client to describe the term. At some point, after teaching what hypnosis is and is not, you will show the client a responsiveness exercise (described later). That's your first step toward refocusing their attention from the analytical to the experiential. After the responsiveness exercise, discuss their experience and coach them on how to better bypass the critical faculty. Then move on to the formal induction process and refocus their attention to your instructions. The induction process then refocuses their attention in such a way that they will enter hypnosis.

Since the altered state is natural, refocused attention is basically just distracting the client from whatever could distract them from entering hypnosis. Refocused attention has five components:

- distraction
- fixation
- suggestion
- relaxation
- repetition

The formal induction process, which induces the altered state, is comprised of all five.

Refocusing attention is how you perform the trance induction "ritual." A ritual is something we do that is expected, appropriate, and intended to bring about a certain outcome. For example, when meeting someone for the first time, you may extend your hand with the intention of shaking hands with them. It is then expected and appropriate for them to reach out and grasp and shake your extended hand. This is a ritual. The person who shakes your hand does so, not because you force them or use magical powers on them, but because they choose to participate in the handshaking ritual. The hypnotic induction is also a ritual. The hypnotherapist initiates the ritual by performing a hypnotic induction, in which case it is expected and appropriate for the client to enter into the special state of mind called hypnosis.

Exciting imagination and building positive expectancy are only effective when the hypnotherapist and the client have rapport, and rapport is necessary to gain the focused attention needed for the induction ritual.

To build strong rapport with a client, you need to become very conscious of the meaning conveyed by the words you use when speaking to and about them. Much of hypnotherapy is the skillful use of semantics. In many hypnotherapy books and courses, it is common to see people referred to as "subjects" and spoken of as "susceptible to hypnosis" or "highly suggestible." Such sloppy use of language by careless or poorly trained hypnotists contributes to the very misconceptions about hypnosis we are trying to clear up.

As hypnotherapists, our work is to empower people to heal themselves. To refer to someone as a "subject" implies that they are somehow inferior or under your control. The word susceptible implies weakness. And if you say that someone is highly suggestible, you've all but called them gullible. This is hardly empowering.

Be aware of your language and always speak to and about people in a manner that conveys respect and a sense of equality. I always refer to people I work with as either client or co-hypnotherapist. For those licensed to practice medicine, the word patient may be more appropriate. Instead of words like susceptible and suggestible, use the word responsive. Not only is it more respectful and empowering, it is also more accurate. Inaccurate wording can create the impression that hypnosis is a form of control, and so it naturally creates resistance to the process. I want to be clear that this is not just a matter of personal preference or taste. Effective hypnotherapy is impossible without rapport, and you cannot build rapport through sloppy, disrespectful, or disempowering communication.

Because of the air of power and mystery already surrounding hypnosis, motion pictures, television shows, novels, and even comic strips often use creative license in presenting it, leaving the public with a distorted view of what hypnosis is and what happens in a hypnotic state. These fantastic portrayals have given rise to some common misconceptions, which are important to dispel in order to facilitate the client's positive response to the healing ritual of hypnosis.

The Misconceptions
There are many misconceptions about hypnosis. For example:

- When hypnotized, you are under the control of the hypnotist.
- You could be made to do something that violates your moral code.
- Hypnosis is a truth serum.
- You lose self-control in hypnosis.
- You will not be aware of what is going on around you while in hypnosis.
- You can become stuck or trapped in hypnosis.

Remember, in reality, hypnosis is simply a natural yet altered state of mind in which the critical faculty is bypassed and selective thinking is established.

Over time, I have found that the most effective way to dispel the myths surrounding hypnosis (many of which continue to be perpetuated by the media in fictional portrayals) is to ask the client which misconceptions they're already aware of, and if they miss any, I add to the list. Dave Elman, (1900-1967) one of the pioneering teachers of medical hypnosis, would sometimes avoid this confusion altogether by referring to hypnosis as a form of "medical relaxation" that helps with healing and pain control.

After dispelling the myths and misconceptions about hypnosis, and explaining the model of the triune mind and how hypnotherapy works, we start the session with some exercises for increasing responsiveness. These processes are for educating the client about what hypnosis really is and how they can use their focused imagination for better results.

Exercises To Increase Responsiveness

Following are some simple exercises that can be used in the pre-hypnosis portion of a session to help a client increase their responsiveness to hypnosis. These exercises are done to coach the client on the best way to use their imagination and focused attention to improve their results with hypnosis. They also provide an important opportunity for the hypnotherapist to begin to excite the imagination, build positive expectancy, and, most importantly, build strong rapport. We want to teach the client to do something I call "managing your suggestibility." This is fairly simple, but crucial. One of the most important parts of managing our response to suggestion is to understand that we get more of whatever we focus on. If we focus on problems and the stress they create, we get more stressful problems. If we focus on how difficult a situation is, the difficulty is what we get. On the other hand, if we focus on solutions, we tend to find solutions.

The Lemon Exercise

Just before you start the lemon exercise is a good time to talk about the use of imagination in hypnosis. Because imagination is a function of the subconscious, intentional use of the imagination engages the subconscious. To perform the lemon exercise, start with an actual lemon that has been cut in half. Show it to your client and then take a bite into it and get some of the fresh juice. Notice the look on their face as you do this. Usually they will look surprised, and they may even grimace as if they themselves had bit the lemon.

After observing their reaction, ask them to describe what happened as they watched you take that bite. They often report that their jaw clenched or that they started to salivate. This is very important information, because it indicates response to suggestion by observation. By just observing you bite into the lemon, they responded as if they were actually physically experiencing what they saw. How many times a day do they have a similar reaction to something someone says or something they see that causes a stress response in the body?

To continue the lemon exercise, instruct the client as follows:

> **"Now, (person's name), I want you to close your eyes and imagine, sense, and feel that I am giving you the other half of the lemon. Imagine that you are biting into it and getting some of the juice. Notice what happens in your mouth as you do this."**

Pause for a few moments and then ask about their experience. With this exercise, about nineteen out of twenty people will have some jaw clenching, salivating, or even a sour taste in their mouth. While this is a very simple exercise, its ramifications are vast. Take this opportunity to point out that, although they did not consciously make their salivary glands secrete saliva, consciously tense their jaw muscles, or consciously make their taste buds perceive a sour taste, all of these things happened. It was all taken care of by their subconscious mind responding to their creative thought and imagination. You'll be showing them how, by using this power of creative thought and imagination, they create these real physical responses in the lemon exercise. They can also use this creative power of the mind to heal their body.

With this exercise, you have demonstrated the principle of suggestion by observation, introduced the idea of managing suggestibility. You have also shown the client that when they involve themselves in the hypnotic instructions, their body responds. This is part of exciting the imagination, establishing belief, and creating positive expectancy. Their response to this exercise is influenced by the level of rapport you have, and the degree to which they involve themselves in the exercise, as well as what kind of subconscious lemon juice associations they make.

The Finger Clamp Exercise

Another great exercise for increasing responsiveness is the finger clamp. Here we invite the client to imagine a clamp that will push their index fingers together (see photo). This exercise requires only willingness and imagination. In preparation for the exercise, make sure that they understand what a clamp looks like, that it has a mechanism to gently tighten it, and that the clamp will only tighten enough to press the fingers tightly together, but not so much that it would hurt the fingers.

To perform the finger clamp exercise, instruct the client as follows:

> "Alright, (person's name), put your palms together, lace your fingers and cross your thumbs. Now separate your index fingers and spread them apart. With your eyes open, imagine that the clamp we talked about before we began is now positioned to push your fingers together. Now imagine, sense, and feel that the clamp starts to tighten slowly, and it begins pushing your fingers gently together. Because you are thinking about the clamp, the clamp is now pushing your index fingers together."

Pause a few seconds.

> "Pushing and moving the fingers together now."

Pause a few seconds.

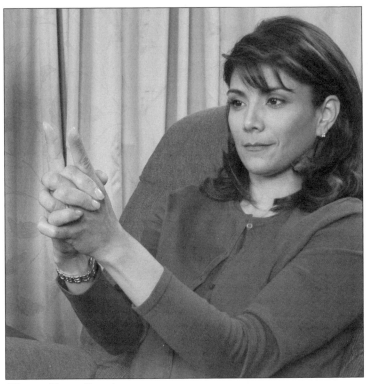

Finger Clamp Exercise

"Gently and easily the index fingers are coming together. The clamp is pushing and pushing the fingers together. Just let it happen."

Wait until the index fingers have come together and touched, then continue:

"Good. You've got it. Now I will remove the clamp and you can separate your hands and tell me about your experience."

Practice this exercise yourself. You will find that, even without an imaginary clamp, when you separate the index fingers, they will naturally want to come back to the neutral, upright position. That's the action of the ligaments and tendons pulling the fingers back together. So if the client's fingers don't come back to at least parallel with each other, that is a clear indication that they are actively fighting the process. Since the clamp they're fighting is only in their imagination, that means they're fighting against themselves. The most common reason for this is that they want to prove that they are in control. Now that they have proof, you can point out that when they were asked to imagine a clamp pushing their fingers together, what they really imagined was their fingers holding a clamp open. This proves that they can maintain control, and that they always get what they focus on. Now you're going to be teaching them a new level of control—control of their thinking and imaginative processes. Learning to be in control of their thinking is what will enable them to heal themselves.

The Balloons and Bucket Exercise

To begin the balloons and bucket exercise, tell the client that you are going to ask them to imagine holding a heavy bucket of wet sand in their right hand and strings attached to a bunch of helium balloons in their left hand. The right arm will then be pulled down by the weight of the bucket while the left arm is lifted up by the pull of the balloons.

> "Put your arms out in front of you. Turn your left hand so the thumb is pointing up and your right hand so the palm is up. Now I will count to three, and when I do, just close your eyes and follow my instructions. One, two, three. Close your eyes. Now, (person's name), imagine the bucket of heavy wet sand. I'm giving it to you now."

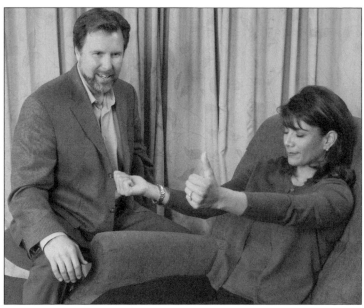

Starting position for Balloon and Bucket Exercise

Gently touch their right palm for a second as if to place the bail of the bucket in the hand, then continue.

> "And because the sand is so heavy, it begins to pull your hand down toward the ground now. The bucket is heavy and pulling the hand down now."

Pause a few seconds.

> "And now here are the strings that are attached to the bunch of balloons."

Gently touch their left hand for a second as if to place the strings in the hand.

> "There are so many balloons that they pull your left hand up, and up, and up toward the ceiling. Imagine

and sense the color of the balloons lifting and lifting your hand up and up."

Pause a few seconds.

"All the while, the bucket of sand is getting heavier and heavier, pulling that hand down, and down... And on the other side, the balloons are lifting and lifting and lifting..."

Wait until client's arms have moved up and down respectively, then continue.

"Wonderful. Now freeze your arms and open your eyes and see where they are."

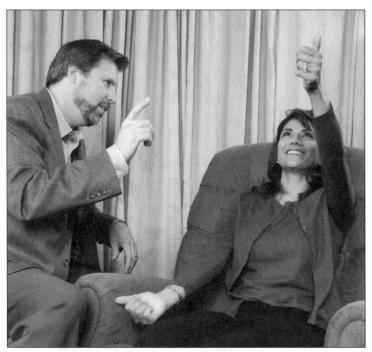

Ending position for Balloon and Bucket Exercise

After they look at their arm positions to see their response, they can put the bucket down and let the balloons go. Then ask them to tell you about their experience.

The Swing Sway Exercise

In the swing sway exercise, you will clearly discover how much rapport you are building as well as how responsive to suggestion the client is becoming. You will ask the client to stand up straight and imagine that they are as stiff as an oak board—completely rigid from head to toe. Then you will rock them a few inches back and forth to see how rigid they have become. Note in the photo how my legs are positioned for stability and my hands are positioned for appropriate touch. Describe the exercise before doing it.

> "(Person's name), what I want you to do this time is stand up straight. Now make your body stiff and rigid. So stiff and rigid, it is as if it were an oak board. Now close your eyes and imagine an oak board, and because you do, every muscle and joint in your body is becoming stiff and rigid. Everything from your head right down to your ankles."

Pause a few seconds.

> "Now your body is so stiff and rigid… As I rock you gently, your body becomes even more stiff and rigid."

Carefully push them about two inches forward and then backward. Do that once or twice, checking that they have made themselves like a board. Then bring them back to the normal upright position and continue.

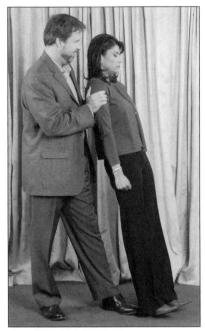
Swing Sway Exercise

"Very good. Now let go of the image and return your body to its normal flexibility and open your eyes."

In this exercise, keep in mind that you are responsible for their balance. Always maintain contact with them so that they feel safe and you can sense if they start to fall over. With a highly responsive client with whom you have excellent rapport, they will become so rigid they may fall over without your assistance. That's just what you want—the highly responsive, excellent rapport part, not the falling.

Debriefing the Responsiveness Exercises

After each exercise, ask the client to talk about their experience. This is an excellent opportunity to debunk misconceptions when they arise. For instance, if they say, "I was waiting for 'it' to happen," meaning, "I just closed my eyes and waited for you to put the spell on me and move my hands by remote control," that's the misconception that they are under the control of the hypnotist. This is a good time to talk about how hypnosis is a team effort in which they are the "co-operator." Explain that you can only teach them what to do with their mind to create healing—you cannot do it for them. That's their job.

Another common report is, "As I listened to your instructions, I was wondering if 'it' would work." Here's a fantastic teaching opportunity! First, you get to explain one of the essential rules of the mind: we get what we focus on. If they are focused on wondering, that is what they get—the experience of wondering; not the lemon flavor, closing fingers, lifting arm, or rigid body. In the same way, if they are wondering if their chemotherapy will work, that may be just what they get—wondering instead of healing. It is far more effective to focus on the chemotherapy working.

Next we get to talk about the "it" word. People new to hypnosis often use this word "it," as in the above case of wondering if "it" would work. The misconception is that the hypnosis is like a pill, and when we take it, it does the work for us. The mistake is in thinking that either the hypnotherapist or the hypnosis will be doing the healing work. Medical hypnotherapy emphasizes self-empowerment. *While we refer to this as medical hypnotherapy, it is not the practice of medicine. These techniques are completely self-help.* We coach and train the client to establish positive beliefs, at the subconscious level, about their body's self-healing capacity. This in turn activates the inherent healing intelligence within them. Ultimately it is the client who does the work of healing. Basically, there is no "it." There's just the client and their mind. We don't inject "it" into them, we don't pour "it" on them, or have them ingest "it."

To help my clients with the "it" word, and the misconception that comes with it, I usually have them try changing the word "it" to "subconscious," or perhaps "mind." This is more accurate and empowering. The sentence then goes something like this: "I was waiting for my subconscious to lift my arm." Now that is something we can work with and coach. At that point I might say something like: "Alright, now here is what I want you to do next time. Instead of waiting for your subconscious to respond, just focus on imagining the suggested imagery as vividly as you possibly can. Involve yourself in the imagery more. Sense it, feel it, and make it real for yourself. That will make a clear impression on your mind, and every impression made on the mind has its physical expression."

Responsiveness also increases as the client becomes aware of their own shift into the altered state. Because they may not recognize this shift, even after you have described what hypnosis isn't (in dispelling myths), it can be helpful to point out some of the signs that hypnosis is actually occurring. There are several very obvious signs of hypnosis that are clearly discernable to the hypnotherapist, and some of these will also be detected by the client as you take them through the process.

The Axiomatic Signs of Hypnosis
In the book *Hypnotherapy* by Dave Elman, five axiomatic signs of hypnosis are described. They are: warm skin, reddening of the sclera, eyeballs rolling up toward the forehead, increased lacrimation, and fluttering eyelids. These five signs of hypnosis are important because they allow the trance state to be recognized by noticeable changes in the client's physiology.

As the human nervous system receives the information that the body is safe, it signals the circulatory system to redirect blood to the surface of the skin, including the tiny blood vessels of the white portion of the eyes, known as the sclera. This results in a flushing of the skin and reddening of the sclera as well as an increase in the surface temperature of the skin, all of which can be easily observed. The eyeballs rolling up toward the forehead can be noticed even with the eyelids closed. The profound relaxation and PNS response that occurs when entering the trance state allows the tear ducts to loosen up and release excess fluid onto the surface of the eye and lacrimation is visibly increased. The involuntary fluttering of the eyelids that often occurs is obvious and unmistakable. Elman thought these signs were particularly important because the typical client with no prior knowledge of hypnosis will not be able to fake them.

Other Signs of Hypnosis

In addition to the five axiomatic signs given by Elman, there are other signs of hypnosis. Some of these are noticeable from the outside, and some can only be experienced by the person in hypnosis.

The extraordinary level of relaxation reached in the hypnotic state helps the various systems of the body return to balance, and function more efficiently. The increase of digestive functions that occurs as a result of this often causes the occasional *stomach gurgle*, which can be heard by the hypnotist.

The *hypnotic mask* is observed when the client becomes so very relaxed that all muscular tension in the facial muscles drains away. The resulting lack of any facial expression gives the impression of a mask.

The *hypnotic sigh* is a deep breath with an audible sighing sound made on the exhalation. A great release of tension usually accompanies the hypnotic sigh and it is often a sign that the client is entering into a deeper level of trance.

Deepened respiration often follows the hypnotic sigh. The depth and rate of respiration may begin to resemble those of someone who is asleep, but the hypnotized person is very much awake. Their body is just responding to the feelings of safety and comfort they experience as they enter deeper into hypnotic relaxation. This deeper breathing brings more oxygen into the body and is very rejuvenating.

Most people experience *hyperacuity of the senses.* Their five senses operate at higher levels of sensitivity; therefore, sights, sounds, smells, tastes, and physical sensations are experienced as more vivid and immediate while in the trance state.

Time distortion is often felt during the trance. While an hour passes on the clock, the hypnotized person may have the subjective experience of being in trance for a significantly shorter or longer period of time. When dehypnotized and asked how long they feel they were in trance, they may say it felt like only a few minutes, or that it felt like a few hours.

Trance is a subjective experience, so everyone experiences hypnosis a bit differently. Seldom do two people ever describe their internal experience of hypnosis in exactly the same way.

The Myth of the Special Induction

There is a myth among some hypnotists that there is a special induction method, script, or technique out there—one that has the magical power to induce trance in anybody and heal everything. Of course, no such thing exists. The myth is based on the reality that you and the client together have the power to heal. The misconception is that the healing comes from the hypnotist using some special technique that does all the work. The power and potential to heal has always been within the client. And when the power of the client and your positive intent become allied in the singular cause of transformation, that is when miracles happen.

CHAPTER
3

Methods to Induce Hypnosis

This chapter will teach you some simple methods to induce the hypnotic state. There are countless induction methods, but because this is a book about medical hypnotherapy, I have chosen to focus on those which are most appropriate for working with accelerating healing and controlling pain both in the field and in the clinical hypnotherapist's office.

The Flow of a Hypnosis Session
A hypnotic induction is typically followed by one or more techniques to deepen and test the hypnotic state. For the sake of clarity and brevity, this chapter will present only the inductions themselves, with deepening and testing techniques covered in depth in the next chapter. Full scripts incorporating induction, deepening, testing, and trance termination are provided in the Appendix. These scripts can be used more or less verbatim to conduct actual sessions in the field. As such, they also serve as excellent

examples of how to combine the techniques presented here with those presented in Chapter Four.

A typical hypnosis session begins with an interview to determine what work needs to be done. If it is the first session with a new client, the hypnotist will also explain how hypnosis works, answer questions, debunk myths, and do some responsiveness exercises. The hypnotist then performs an induction, followed by deepening and testing techniques. Once the client is in hypnosis, the hypnotist guides the client through whatever processes are appropriate and then delivers therapeutic suggestions and healing imagery. When the work is complete, the hypnotist terminates the trance and conducts a short interview to get feedback and help the client integrate their experience. At the end of the session, the hypnotist will often assign activities for the client to do on their own to accelerate their progress.

The Fundamental Agreement
The hypnotic induction is really the process of two people entering into an agreement with each other. At the conscious level, the hypnotist agrees to help the client mobilize their inner resources to heal themselves, and the client agrees to actively engage in the process and be the co-operator. This conscious agreement to co-operate in working toward a common goal is the basis of the therapeutic relationship.

Just as crucial as the conscious agreement to co-operate is the agreement that takes place at the subconscious level. This is not an explicit, spoken agreement, but rather a special kind of rapport that develops when certain elements are present in the relationship.

The first and most essential element is readiness for change. A client who is really ready to change may achieve their goal even with an unskilled hypnotist. But if the client is not ready to change, even the most skillful application of hypnotherapy methods may prove fruitless.

In addition to readiness for change, the client must believe that the change they desire is possible for them and that the hypnotist is capable of assisting them with that change. You will need to nurture and develop these attitudes in the client during the pre-hypnosis portion of the session. You can do this in part by relating stories of others who have had success in similar circumstances, through responsiveness exercises, and other overt means, but the most effective method is simply to hold these beliefs yourself. When you have strong faith and belief in yourself, in the methods of hypnosis, and in the client and their ability to heal themselves, your every action will communicate this. The client will sense the calm confidence inside of you and subconsciously respond with their own feeling of confidence and positive expectation. By holding in your mind the image of the client as already healed, you create a field of healing potential in which they too can see healing as a real possibility for themselves.

These elements add up to create a subconscious agreement to succeed. This is the fundamental agreement that underlies all successful hypnotic inductions and processes. This is the magic ingredient that transforms your words and intentions into positive change and healing.

A Competence-Building Secret

For nearly two decades, we have been providing hypnotherapy certification training at the Hypnotherapy Academy of America. The trainees have proved over and over that the quickest way to achieve the level of competence needed is to approach learning the methods with a very special attitude—the beginner's mind. Beginner's mind is an attitude of positive inquiry in which all preconceived notions and skepticism are set aside. It's an attitude of playful exploration, fresh openness, and positive expectation.

The new hypnosis practitioner must approach each session with the intention that the client will respond and experience some positive movement. *What is expected tends to be realized.* Be it a lack of self-confidence or a researcher's skepticism, any attitude that sets up negative expectations will act as a subconscious saboteur. So instead of looking for what is wrong or what does not work, look for what is right and what does work and keep doing more of that. Positive intention is your key to success. When practicing these methods, have fun with them and expect the best.

Modified Elman Two Finger Eye Closure Induction

The first induction we teach in the training is a modified version of Dave Elman's "Two Finger Eye Closure." Elman based this method on the earlier work of French physician and hypnosis pioneer Ambroise Auguste Liebeault (1823-1904). You will find it a rapid induction excellent for use in the private office, hospital emergency department, or medical clinic.

Remember that the way you approach the client is part of the induction. Before beginning with an induction, it is a good idea to get the client's consent to do so by asking something like, "Are you ready for me to hypnotize you now?" or, "I'm going to show you a medical relaxation technique to help you stay calm and relaxed during the procedure. Shall I begin?" When the client answers in the affirmative, not only does it give you permission to proceed, it acts as a kind of pre-suggestion for them, setting up the expectation that whatever you do next will induce the hypnotic state. With this positive expectation working, and with the client's consent, you can then proceed with the induction as follows:

"Begin by finding a spot high on the ceiling to stare at... Now take in a nice, deep breath... Now open your eyes as wide as you can... Take another deep breath, keeping your eyes open wide... Now I'm going to close your eyes with my finger and thumb."

Reach over and gently guide the client's eyes closed with your forefinger and thumb. Your forefinger and thumb should come to rest on the client's cheekbones, with a slight bit of pressure on the eyelids.

"Now relax the eyelid muscles beneath my finger and thumb."

Pause 5 seconds.

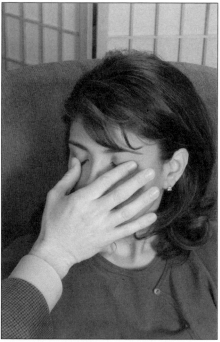

Elman Eye Closure

"Now as I pull away my hand, continue relaxing the eyelids fully and completely. In fact, I want you to relax those eyelids so much that they just won't work."

Pause 5 seconds.

"When you feel that you have relaxed them to the point where they just won't work, nod your head."

Client nods.

"Now go ahead and test them and when you're satisfied that they just won't work, say 'satisfied' out loud."

Client says "Satisfied."

"Now send that relaxation that's around the eyes all the way down through your body, down to the very tips of your toes."

Now the client is in hypnosis and you can move on to deepening and testing techniques, which will be covered in Chapter Four.

Flashlight Induction
The flashlight induction emphasizes the visual fixation component of refocused attention by having the client stare into a penlight. In the 1840's, a physician named James Braid found that he could get patients to enter the hypnotic state by having them stare fixedly at a lantern. At the time, this was a very mysterious finding and was referred to as being "mesmerized," a term coined after Franz Anton Mesmer.

After Braid's discovery, it was believed for a time that only by visual fixation could one enter into the hypnotic trance. We now know that visual fixation is only one of many ways to create the refocused attention necessary to induce hypnosis. This induction works well for both adults and children. As before, begin by asking for the client's consent.

> **"Would you like me to show you an easy way to go into hypnosis so you can feel better?"**

Position the penlight about twelve inches from the client's face and up about 45 degrees above their line of sight. Aim the beam at the tip of the client's nose.

> **"Now look at the light and keep your eyes open while I count backwards from five down to one.**

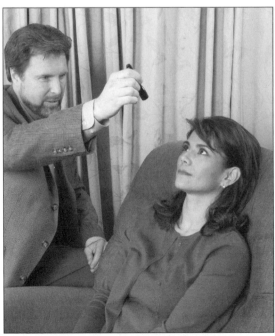

Starting position for Flashlight Induction

When I reach the number one, just close your eyes and you will be in a pleasant state of hypnosis."

As you slowly count backwards (script follows), move the light down towards the client's face in an arc. Keep the beam of light pointed at the tip of the nose throughout the entire movement. By the time you reach the number one, your hand should be at the level of the client's chin, with the beam angled up slightly toward the nose.

Some clients will need more time to relax. With these clients, before counting backwards and descending the penlight, have them first stare at the light as you move it from the centerline to the left about 3 inches. Then have them take a deep breath and exhale as you hold the light to the left of center. After the exhale, move the penlight back to the center, pause there for a couple seconds, then move it to the right of the centerline about 3 inches. Instruct the client to take another deep breath in and exhale while you hold the penlight to the right of center. After the exhale, bring the light back to center and begin the count backwards, moving the penlight down towards the client's face in an arc as described above.

> "Five… Staring at the light takes you into hypnosis, and your eyes automatically become heavy and tired…
>
> Four… Looking at the light, your eyes begin to feel heavy and tired as if sleepy…
>
> Three… Your eyes are getting heavier and heavier. Blinking is hypnosis coming on…
>
> Two… It will feel so good to close your eyes, and relax…

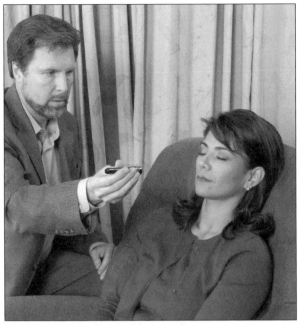

Ending position for Flashlight Induction

One… Just close your eyes down as you drift even deeper and deeper relaxed…"

Move the light away and turn the beam off. The client is now in hypnosis and you can proceed with deepening and testing.

Ideomotor Movement as an Induction

A dominant idea, be it from suggestion or expectation (which is then converted to an autosuggestion), creates involuntary and subconsciously directed motor movement—the transduction of a thought into a biological action. In 1852, physiologist William Carpenter coined the term "ideomotor" to describe this action. This induction makes use of a pendulum to give the client a direct experience of ideomotor movement.

In this induction we invite the client to hold the string or chain of a pendulum between their finger and thumb with their arm straight out in front of them. Then, with their eyes open, we ask them to hold their hand steady and at the same time vividly imagine the pendulum swinging left and right just like a clock's pendulum. This image makes an impression upon the subconscious mind which then creates micro-movements in the client's shoulder and arm that start the pendulum swinging left and right. The more vividly the client imagines the swinging pendulum, the greater the swing of the actual pendulum in their hand, thereby illustrating the principle that what they impress upon their mind will have its physical expression in their body.

There are two key benefits to the use of this induction. First, the client has an actual experience of how a thought creates a physical reaction in their body. And second, since they are the one holding and directing the pendulum, they get to feel more like they are in charge of the induction process. While the client is always ultimately responsible for their responsiveness, the aid of the physical or mechanical adjunct of the pendulum adds to the experience. Also, the client has their eyes open for a good part of the induction and that seems to hold them in the experience more.

This induction works well with highly analytical clients. People who are very analytical often complain that the slower inductions that include progressive relaxation, guided imagery, mental confusion and so on, "don't work." When I interview these people, I usually find that they were busy analyzing the induction, and therefore not experiencing it. Remember, they get what they focus on. Analysis is a conscious mind function, and engaging the conscious mind reduces access to the subconscious.

The fact that a thought of an action will be transduced into actual biological action is at the very foundation of psychoneuroimmunology and medical hypnotherapy. This induction provides a direct experience of this fact that not only amazes the client, but also becomes a powerful metaphor that empowers them in their own healing process. Take time before and after using this method to talk with your client about the implications. Explain that in the same way they were able to get the pendulum swinging just by picturing it, by seeing themselves as fully healed they can get their body to do what it needs to make that happen.

Begin by approaching the client this way:

"I want to show you a hypnosis method that also teaches you how to direct the power of your subconscious mind. Shall we begin?"

When the client responds in the affirmative, give them the pendulum and have them hold it out in front of them between their first finger and thumb.

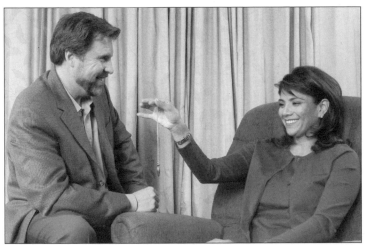

Starting position for Pendulum Induction

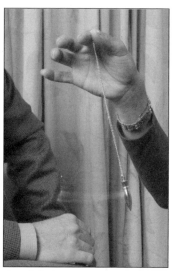

Pendulum swinging

"Now I want you to stare directly at the pendulum and hold it as steady as possible. As you look at the pendulum, vividly imagine it swinging side to side just like a clock pendulum swings side to side. (Person's name), picture the pendulum swinging side to side. Just use the power of your mind to move the pendulum. Want it to happen… See it happening… Then it happens…"

Pause for about 5 seconds.

"That's it, just imagine the pendulum swinging side to side, and it swings side to side. Just watch what happens to the pendulum."

Watch the pendulum yourself, and be encouraging as the movement begins. Some people will picture the pendulum swinging so successfully that the movement begins in only 5 to 10 seconds. Others may take 15 to 20 seconds to get some movement.

After the client has the pendulum swinging from side to side, simply by visualizing it, have them change the direction of the movement so that the pendulum swings either in a circle or toward and away from them.

> "Good, you are doing very well. Now I want you to change the movement of the pendulum so that it swings either in a circle or toward and away from you. Once you've chosen the new movement, just picture and vividly imagine the pendulum swinging in that new direction. Just use the power of your mind to move the pendulum. Want it to happen... See it happening... Then it happens."

Occasionally the client will need a little more guidance in order to get their mind focused on the correct imagery to bring about the desired movement in the pendulum. You can help by repeating and embellishing the instructions for them.

After the client has the pendulum swinging in the new direction, you can be assured they have established contact with their subconscious and it has become responsive to their instruction. They are putting themselves into hypnosis. Now it is time to deepen the experience. Speak in a calm, melodious voice as you give the following instructions:

> "Now as you watch the pendulum, let your arm and eyes begin to get heavy and tired feeling...
>
> Notice what happens as your arm gets even heavier now. Your eyes are on the pendulum, and your arm is getting so heavy, that it begins to slowly pull down, towards your lap...

> That's right, and as soon as the pendulum touches your lap, your eyes close and you'll be in a pleasant state of hypnosis…
>
> Your arm is getting heavier and heavier, pulling down… down… down to your lap. You may notice that even your eyes are feeling heavy… heavy… heavy and tired…
>
> As soon as the pendulum touches your lap, your eyes close and you are in that pleasant state of hypnosis…"

The pendulum touches their lap and their eyes close. This is an excellent time to begin conditioning the client to use self-hypnosis. Reach over, gently touch the client's forehead with a couple fingers as you say the following:

> "Sleep now. When I say, 'sleep now' I'm not referring to the kind of sleep you sleep at night. I'm referring to this pleasant hypnotic state where you have released stress and tension and you are relaxed. Whenever you want to go into hypnosis, you can use your pendulum and when it touches your lap, just say 'sleep now' and you easily and immediately go into a pleasant hypnotic state. Not because I say so, but because it's the nature and ability of your subconscious mind to do so."

Remove your hand. The client is now in hypnosis and you can proceed with deepening and testing.

Touching the forehead complies with the limits of appropriate touch and assists by signaling the nervous system to link these instructions to the feeling of hypnosis. In general, a kinesthetic signal strengthens the verbal suggestion.

Boyne's Hand Press Method for Instantaneous Induction
I was first taught this method by Gil Boyne and I find it exceptionally useful for three reasons. First, if you only have a short time to induce and develop a therapeutic trance, this is the induction of choice. Second, if the client is overly analytical, this induction bypasses the critical faculty so fast that they don't have the time to analyze their experience, they just have their experience. Third, the client who is more kinesthetic and auditory than visual will have a better response to this instantaneous induction because it engages them in a way that is more familiar to them. For kinesthetic and auditory people, the more typical guided imagery inductions can be very frustrating.

This induction makes use of the "startle command" technique. When a person is even slightly startled they experience a momentary loss of certainty. At that point, all analytical thinking stops until a decision is made about how to react. In such a situation, as a kind of decision-making shortcut, humans and other social animals will look to others to find out what to do. That means that a startled person has a moment in which their critical faculty is wide open, making them very responsive to decisive suggestion.

Imagine it's 10,000 years ago. We are both cavemen and we are out hunting for the clan's dinner. All of a sudden we hear a deep growling sound come from the nearby bushes. We both startle and freeze in our tracks. I, being the more experienced of the two of us, have heard this sound before, and I have seen the bear that makes it. I grunt at you, "Bear! Run!" and then I bolt. Now one of two things is going to happen—either you will analyze the situation or you will run. For your sake, I hope you run, because if you stop to analyze the situation, you are one dead caveman.

The startle command technique consists of startling the client to create a moment of openness and uncertainty and then immediately giving them the clear and decisive instruction "SLEEP!" The sleep command is delivered in a sharp and commanding tone, conveying a sense of certainty and urgency. This technique should only be attempted when the hypnotist and client have excellent rapport and the client sees the hypnotist as a confident authority in hypnosis. While only slightly startling, it is not to be used with cardiac patients. Begin as follows:

"Would you like to learn a way to go into hypnosis instantly?"

Client responds in the affirmative. Hold your hand out palm up and say the following with a firm, strong voice.

"Okay, put your hand on mine. Now start pushing down on my hand. I want you to press firmly."

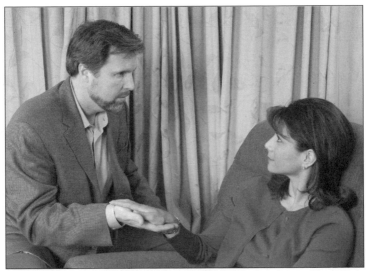

Beginning position for Hand Press Induction

Point to your eye with your free hand as you say the following.

"Now I want you to look directly into my eye."

While client is looking into your eye, continue.

"Look into my eye and go into hypnosis. As you look into my eye, your eyes start to get heavy and tired. Each time they blink, that's hypnosis coming on. Eyes are getting heavy, droopy, and drowsy."

Move your non-pressing hand very slowly toward the client's face to non-verbally communicate that you want them to close their eyes and continue with the following.

"Now eyes closing… closing… closing… Eyes getting heavier, tired and closing now. Closing them."

The moment the eyes close and stay closed for about one or two seconds, immediately strengthen your voice and deliver the sleep command as you simultaneously jerk your hand out from underneath the client's hand so that they lurch forward slightly. A slight loss of equilibrium helps to induce the trance. At the very moment you jerk your hand back, deliver the startle command.

"SLEEP!"

Then gently push the client's head back to the recliner chair and rock their head from side to side about an inch or two for deepening the trance. If the client is not sitting or lying such that they have a surface to support their head, you can also lean their head forward so that their forehead is cradled by your hand and rock it back and forth that way.

> "Now, you are going deep into hypnosis. Neck muscles relaxing and letting go. Let me gently rock your head side to side while you go deeper and deeper. Your neck muscles are becoming loose and limp and relaxed now. When I use the word sleep, I am not referring to the kind of sleep you sleep at night. I am referring to this hypnotic state you are now experiencing."

After slowly rocking the head side to side three or four times, move on to deepening and testing.

Sequential Imagery as an Induction

The use of imagery as an induction is most useful for clients who are visually dominant. See Chapter Six for a method you can use to determine if your client is more visual, kinesthetic, or auditory before using this method. As a general rule, always check that the imagery you will be using is appropriate to use with the client by giving a brief example of the elements of the imagery in the script. If you guide the client in imagining themselves relaxing by the poolside and they nearly drowned in a pool when they were a child, they're more likely to have a fight-or-flight reaction than go into hypnosis.

Sequential imagery as an induction involves both hemispheres of the brain by including numeric sequences with vivid images. The left hemisphere becomes involved with the numbers and the right hemisphere with the pictures. While you can be creative with the setting, common ones include stairs, elevators, and escalators. I will provide you with an example of a sequential imagery induction I have used for years. This script includes the use of a set of steps that lead to an ocean beach.

After clearing the elements of the imagery with the client, continue with the following. Speak in a slow and melodious voice.

> "Please take a good, long, deep breath and close your eyes. Now make yourself comfortable and prepare for a very enjoyable journey. Imagine you are outside. It's a bright, sunny day, and there is a gentle breeze. Imagine you are standing at the top of a set of ten steps that lead down to a warm and inviting beach. The steps are very sturdy because they are set in the earth. Put a hand-rail on both sides of the stairs. Look at the steps. There are ten steps and they are numbered as well. The top step has the number ten on it, the next step has a nine on it, and so on all the way down to the last step, which has the number one on it. The last step, which is at the bottom, is on the beach.
>
> In a moment I will begin counting backwards. As I do, vividly imagine that you are slowly walking down the steps. Go down one step with each number I speak. With each step you will go deeper and deeper into hypnotic relaxation. On the number one you will be on the last step and eager to step off into the warm sand.
>
> Alright. Number ten… Imagine, sense, and feel yourself step down, going down deeper into hypnosis.
>
> Number nine… Step down. Going down deeper, deeper, and deeper relaxed with each step you imagine yourself taking. Imagine the warm breeze is becoming real for you. You imagine what the smell of the salt air would be like.

Number eight... See the number eight written on the step and step down, going deeper and deeper relaxed.

Number seven... Step down. Going down deeper, deeper, and deeper relaxed with each step you imagine yourself taking. The big blue sky has a few clouds in it, and if you like, you can hear the call of seagulls now as you get closer to the bottom of the stairs.

Number six... Imagine, sense, and feel that you are stepping down onto the sixth step, and you are going deeper and deeper relaxed.

Five... Step down. Put yourself halfway down the steps. You are halfway to the warm sandy beach at the bottom of the stairs."

Now start slowing your speech pattern slightly.

"Four... Step down to the fourth step. And go down deeper, deeper, and deeper relaxed with each step you imagine yourself taking.
Number three... You are almost there on the beach.

Two... Down, down, down, deeper, deeper, deeper.
One... Step down onto the last step. In a moment you will step down onto the beach and go deeper into hypnosis. You're relaxing deeply and that feels good. Okay, please imagine you are barefoot now and then step off into the warm sand.

As you step into the sand you sink down about an inch into the soft, warm granules of sand. Put a lounge chair with a bright umbrella over it a few feet in front of you. Walk over to the lounge chair and get in it. The shade produced by the umbrella makes this place just the right temperature for you. Out in the distance you see the gentle ocean waves lapping back and forth on the sand. Here in this place of perfect serenity your subconscious mind is open and receptive to the beneficial ideas we spoke about before hypnosis."

The client is now in a profoundly relaxed state of hypnosis and you can proceed with accelerated healing and pain control techniques, suggestion therapy, and other healing imagery.

Terminating the Trance

Whenever you use a hypnotic induction you will need to perform a trance termination to help the client return to their normal everyday awareness, regardless of whether or not the client "feels" like they were in a trance. Terminating the trance is usually done by counting from one up to five while giving a series of suggestions to the client to bring themselves out of hypnosis, feeling good in every way and acting on the positive suggestions delivered during the session. If the client went very deep into hypnosis, extend the count to ten to allow them more time to make the transition. When counting someone out of hypnosis it is important to change your voice tone and tempo. As the client transitions from hypnosis into their everyday state of alert awareness, energize your voice and quicken the pace of your speech. Intersperse the instructions with suggestions that reinforce whatever positive changes the client made during the session. You can also include empowering suggestions that affirm their ability to successfully practice self-hypnosis and have an increasingly profound experience with every hypnosis session. Here's an example of a typical five-count trance termination.

> "Alright, (person's name), in a moment I will count from one up to five. As I do, bring yourself out of hypnosis and bring with you all the peace and comfort you are now experiencing. When I say the number five, you will then open your eyes, stretch, and smile, and be fully alert.
>
> One… Slowly, calmly, and gently bring yourself up and out of hypnosis. All the good, comfortable sensations stay with you as you come out of hypnosis.
>
> Two… Each muscle in your body is loose, limp, and relaxed. You feel good. Your body continues to heal itself rapidly now. Each and every time you practice hypnosis, you respond more profoundly, going deeper into relaxation with every session.
>
> Three… As you bring yourself up and out of hypnosis you feel wonderful in every way. You are emotionally calm and serene, physically at ease, and mentally clear and alert. You look forward to practicing hypnosis again.
>
> Four… Preparing to open your eyes on the next number. In a moment, when you open your eyes, you are fully alert.
>
> Five… Eyes open now. Stretch, smile, and notice how good you feel."

Patter Patter Patter

Patter is the repetition, variation, and embellishment of hypnotic instructions to fit the needs of the client. Some people will need more time and guidance to respond to your instructions, others will need less. Learning to use patter correctly is what will give you the flexibility to adapt to each client.

Let's use the flashlight induction as an example. At the end of the flashlight induction, you count backward from five while descending the light and giving suggestions that their eyes will get heavy and tired and then close when you reach the number one. A highly responsive client may start to close their eyes at number four and you would then shorten the script to something like, "Four, closing down. Three, two, and one. Eyelids closed." That's using less patter. A less responsive client may not have even blinked by the time you get to three, so you would want to start repeating: "Eyelids getting heavy and tired… heavy and tired," varying: "Slowly closing down, eyelids closing, closing shut," and embellishing: "Feeling almost as if small weights are pulling your eyelids down, making them so heavy." The skillful use of patter requires only that you pay careful attention to the client and how they are responding to what you say so that you can adapt to fit their needs.

CHAPTER 4

Deepening and Testing Techniques

This chapter presents a variety of techniques for deepening and testing the hypnotic state. Deepening and testing techniques follow the induction. These techniques further open the critical faculty of the conscious mind by refocusing the client's attention on their internal experience and guiding them "deeper" into their subconscious level of awareness.

Deepening techniques create the physical and mental relaxation required for accelerating healing processes and pain control. Physical relaxation is experienced as the absence of muscular tension, so many of the techniques focus on helping the client to relax their body completely. Mental relaxation is experienced as the absence of spontaneous thought, so other techniques focus on developing a clear and relaxed mind. The client's subconscious is most receptive to suggestions of healing or pain control when both types of relaxation have been achieved.

Hypnotic tests provide feedback for both the client and the hypnotherapist about how responsive to suggestion the client has become. The tests provide the client with a physical experience of their responsiveness by suggesting, for example, that the client's eyelids are locked shut and cannot be opened or that their arm is locked straight and cannot be bent. When the client then tries to open their eyes or bend their arm and finds that they are unable to do so, they consciously realize that they are in trance and that their subconscious is successfully responding to suggestion. When this realization occurs, the client is able to stop wondering and trust the process, which helps them relax more and respond more profoundly to subsequent suggestions. This is referred to as "deepening by realization."

When you really boil it all down, the point of the induction, deepening, and testing is to assist the client in developing a responsive subconscious—a subconscious that responds to new and beneficial programming. The deepening and testing techniques help the client learn to communicate with and direct their subconscious creative energies. With this communication comes a special quality of communion between the mind and the body that is valuable in hypnotic pain control, self-healing, and the prevention of stress-provoked "dis-ease." Deepening and testing give the client fairly simple methods to practice this kind of communication.

Deepening Techniques
Arm Drop
The arm drop is a simple deepening technique. It serves two purposes. First, when you lift your client's arm you can check for relaxation. When the arm is heavy and loose, you know that the client is responding to your suggestion. Second, the client becomes aware of the physical sensation of their relaxation. It is crucial that the client be able to distinguish between the feeling of tension and the feeling

Deepening and Testing Techniques 77

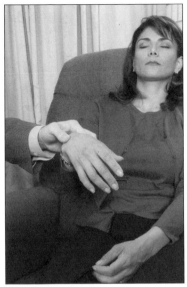

Arm Drop

of relaxation. This allows the client to internally mark the feeling of relaxation so they can return to it much more easily in the future. Begin as follows:

> "In a moment I am going to lift your arm up and drop it like this."

Lift the client's arm up about six inches, gripping it either by the wrist or by the thumb, and then gently place it back down. Be conscious of anatomy and appropriate touch.

> "When I do, just let your arm be loose, limp, and heavy. Let me have the full weight of your arm and let me do all the lifting. And when I drop the arm, just let it plop down. I will then say the words 'sleep deeper.' 'Sleep deeper' is your signal to double your relaxation. Alright, I'm going to pick up your arm now."

Now lift the client's arm just as you demonstrated. Notice whether or not they have responded to your suggestions to relax their arm and let you do all the lifting. If you notice that they are still tense or that they are helping you lift the arm, you can gently wiggle the arm while using patter to help them relax it completely. When the arm is completely relaxed, drop it and say:

"Sleep deeper and double your relaxation."

For a person who is in need of pain erasure, you can embellish the arm drop by suggesting increased comfort with the hand plopping down. If, for example, they had pain in their right leg, you could embellish the arm drop with something like, "Now as your hand plops down, double your relaxation. And because you are doubling your relaxation, you feel more and more comfort moving into your right leg now."

Head Roll
The head roll relaxes the neck muscles, which in turn helps the client relax all the muscles of the head and shoulders. In the script, you suggest that the neck muscles become relaxed while you gently rock the head back and forth. The hand on the forehead and the gentle rocking helps to refocus their attention on the suggested task. Clients often report how combining the tactile with the verbal suggestion really makes it easier for them to keep their mind focused on developing relaxation.

To perform the head roll, place your hand on the client's forehead and rock their head gently back and forth as you say the following.

"Just let your neck muscles relax and go loose and limp. Neck muscles relaxing and letting go with

each gentle rocking motion of your head back and forth. Going deeper and deeper into hypnosis. Your neck muscles are becoming loose and limp and relaxed now. Just send that relaxation throughout your entire body and go two times deeper into hypnosis now."

Progressive Relaxation

Progressive relaxation consists of slowly releasing all unnecessary tension from the body, region by region. This can be achieved by either direct suggestion or the combination of suggestion and physically tensing and relaxing the muscular regions of the body. It can be used as an induction, or for deepening. In the following example, because the client is already in hypnosis, we simply use direct suggestions and the client responds quite well.

In our normal, everyday state of awareness, our attention is focused externally. As long as we're focused on external

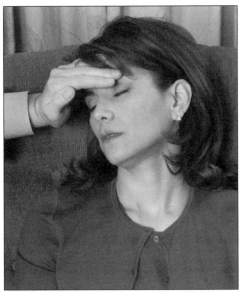

Head Roll

circumstances, the mind and body maintain a certain degree of tension. By intentionally turning the attention inward and focusing on relaxing during the progressive relaxation process, the natural vigilance of the mind is relaxed and the body is able to let go of muscular tension completely. Begin as follows:

> "Now, to become more deeply relaxed and even more responsive to positive healing ideas, begin to relax all the muscles in your scalp. You are safe, and you begin to feel a great wave of peace flow over you. Imagine a warm, relaxing feeling moving into your neck. Think about all the neck muscles becoming loose and limp."

Pause a few seconds to allow the client to think about and experience the relaxation.

> "Now slowly and gently move the warm relaxation into your shoulders and down into your arms. Just use the power of your imagination. Just imagine the muscles turning loose and limp and relaxing more and more. Your shoulders, arms, and hands are becoming pleasantly warm and relaxed."

Pause a few seconds.

> "Move the comfortable relaxing sensation down your back now. Imagine, sense, and feel that you are sending the warm relaxing energy into all the muscles of your back. Picture all the back muscles loosening and relaxing now."

Pause a few seconds.

"You are becoming more deeply relaxed and at peace now. Send the warm, relaxing sensation down into your hips and legs. Slowly, easily, and gently, imagine the relaxing sensation melting away any tension as the warm, relaxing, comfortable feeling moves down, down, down into your legs."

Pause a few seconds.

"Send the relaxing sensation down past your ankles now and into your feet. Your feet and toes are becoming warm and relaxed and comfortable now, and your subconscious mind is open and will act upon positive healing ideas. Just being in this hypnotic relaxation is healing for you, (person's name). Enjoy this pleasant time as your body restores itself to perfect health."

Warm Light

The body holds and reflects our thoughts, so the quality of our thoughts dictates what the body feels. With the warm light deepening method, the client imagines a warm and restoring sunlight shining down on them. Light brings life and warmth. By filling the mind with this quality of thought, the body has a respite from holding stress thoughts and is filled with thoughts that create warmth and comfort. When the body becomes warm, it is a sign that the parasympathetic nervous system is becoming active, and you can be assured that other beneficial body functions are being promoted as well.

In the warm light deepening method you also invite the client to roll their eyes up slightly as you describe the imagery. In many cases this helps to make visualization easier and more vivid.

Begin as follows:

"Now roll your eyes up slightly toward your forehead. Like a beam of sunlight, imagine, sense, and feel a beautiful, warm, relaxing light descending upon you from above. This light brings you a peaceful, relaxing feeling. Now imagine this warm and relaxing energy moving down into your scalp. Down into your neck and shoulders. Feel the relaxing energy moving in, and you're relaxing more and more.

This warm and relaxing energy is moving down into the arms, hands, and fingers. Pure, white light restoring you to perfect health. Relaxing warm light.

And now imagine this energy moving into your chest and abdomen and all through your back.

With each easy breath you breathe, the warm light is healing you, and restoring your vitality. Breathing easily and relaxing the body and mind. Feel yourself relaxing more as you imagine the warm, relaxing light moving down through your hips and into your legs. Warm and relaxing stillness. Warm and relaxing stillness from the top of your head all the way down into your ankles, your feet and toes."

Ten Count for Deepening

The monotonous presentation of an idea that does not require a lot of conscious analysis is an effective means of deepening the hypnotic state in most cases. By this time in the hypnosis experience, the client's critical faculty is already opening. They may still analyze what you are saying for the first few numbers, but eventually they will become bored with the monotony and just disengage even more.

> "In a moment I will count from ten down to one. With each number that I count, you will relax more and more. As I count, imagine moving through a passageway to a safe and peaceful place. Make it as vivid as you would like. When I reach the number one, just be in that peaceful, pleasant place, feeling totally relaxed.
>
> Just relax yourself more with each number that I count. And when I reach the number one, you will be ten times deeper. When I reach the number one, I will say the words 'sleep deeper.' That will be your signal to imagine yourself settling in that safe and wonderful place, feeling good in every way. Maybe a meadow, or a beach, or perhaps a garden. Anywhere you love being. A place that you would like to come back to and visit again and again."

Now start counting slowly. Time the repetitive phrase "deeper relaxed" to their exhale, implicitly connecting the idea of relaxing deeper and releasing tension to the release of air from the lungs. Speak in a relaxing tone and slow your rate of speech as you count down.

> "Ten… Deeper relaxed.
>
> Nine… Deeper, deeper, deeper relaxed.
>
> Eight… Down, down, down, deeper relaxed.
>
> Seven… Deeper, deeper, deeper relaxed.

> Six... Imagine moving toward that peaceful, pleasant place, and because you are, you relax even more.
>
> Five... Down, down, down, deeper relaxed.
>
> Four... Deeper, deeper, deeper relaxed.
>
> Three... Getting closer to that peaceful, pleasant place, and because you are, you relax even more.
>
> Two... Down, down, down, deeper relaxed.
>
> One... Sleep deeply. (Person's name), enjoy being in your peaceful, pleasant place now. Rest here, feeling safe and completely comfortable, free and at peace with all creation while I am quiet."

Elman Eye Closure

Because the eye closure method so perfectly refocuses the client's attention on their internal experience by putting all their attention on the structure of the eyelid muscles, it may be used as both an induction and a deepening method. It's a good idea to start with smaller muscle groups and go on to larger ones after the skill of intentionally releasing tension is developed. Because the musculature that opens and closes the eyelids is a small group and easy to isolate, it's a good place to start. Begin as follows:

> "Now (person's name), put all of your attention on your eyelids. Relax your eyelid muscles completely. Relax the upper eyelids and the lower eyelids fully and completely. Relax the eyelids so much that they just won't work."

Pause for 5 seconds.

> "When you have relaxed them so much that you are sure that they just won't work, nod your head."

Client nods.

> "In that case, go ahead and test them. Test them hard, and find that they just won't work."

Give the client a few seconds to try to open their eyes unsuccessfully, then continue with the following:

> "Wonderful. Stop trying now and notice how good that feels. Now send that relaxation that you have in and around your eyes all throughout your body, from the top of your head down to the tips of your toes."

Repeated Eye Closure

Repeated eye closure accomplishes two important goals. First, it is a repeated induction, which, because the effects of hypnosis are accumulative and progressive, tends to compound the hypnotic state. Second, the client has a direct experience of being in control and in charge of the deepening process. This was one of Elman's favorite deepening methods, no doubt because the dynamic relationship of your suggestion for deepening and the client's co-operation is extremely effective. Begin as follows:

> "In a moment I'll ask you to open and close your eyes. Each time I have you open and close your eyes, your physical relaxation will grow twice as great. Just want that to happen and it will happen. Alright, open your eyes… Now close your eyes and let your physical

relaxation double. Just let go and feel your body relaxing. Let that feeling of relaxation go all through your body, (person's name)."

Pause a few seconds to allow the client to deepen their relaxation.

"In a moment I'll ask you to open and close your eyes again. And again, when you close your eyes, double this physical relaxation. Okay, open your eyes... Now close your eyes. Close them and you're going way down... deeper... deeper relaxed. Send the relaxation all throughout your body now."

Pause a few seconds to allow the client to deepen their relaxation.

"Good. And now let's do that one more time. Go ahead and open your eyes... And just let them close down and double your physical relaxation again. Really letting go. Going down... down... deeper relaxed. Send that feeling throughout your whole body now."

Elman's Disappearing Numbers

After years of experimentation, Elman discovered that when the client achieves true mental relaxation they can best control pain. As physical relaxation is the absence of tension, mental relaxation is the absence of spontaneous thought—thoughts like, "How much is this going to hurt?" The untrained and undisciplined mind acts somewhat like a drunken monkey. It will grab hold of any thought and play with it. By teaching the disappearing numbers technique, you are showing the client how to gain control of their mind. It is taming the "monkey mind." When they can control their mind, they can do miraculous things like control their perception and therefore, their experience of their medical procedures. This technique is only effective after physical relaxation has already been achieved.

Begin as follows:

> "Now that you are physically relaxed, I want to show you how to mentally relax. You see, (person's name), when you relax your mind, you can do anything. We want your mind to be just as relaxed as your body. So, when I tell you to, I want you to start counting backward from 100 out loud. For each number, starting at 100, first say the number out loud. Then I want you to double your mental relaxation as you make the number disappear completely from your mind. You'll say the number, then relax it out, sending it out of your mind. Then, when that number is gone, say, 'Faded away.' Then say the next number, and relax it out of your mind, and so on. By the time you reach 97, you will be so mentally relaxed that all numbers will have completely disappeared from your mind temporarily.
>
> Alright, begin by saying, '100.' Then double your relaxation and send it out of your mind. When it's completely gone from your mind, say, 'Faded away.'"

Client says, "100."

> "Make it disappear as you double your mental relaxation. When it's completely gone from your mind, say, 'Faded away.'"

Client says, "Faded away."

"Now say the next number."

Client says, "99."

"Make it disappear as you double your mental relaxation. When it's completely gone from your mind, say, 'Faded away.'"

Client says, "Faded away."

"Good. Say the next number."

Client says, "98."

"Send it out of your mind."

Client says, "Faded away."

"Good. Just continue doubling your mental relaxation."

Client says, "97."

"Double your mental relaxation."

Client says, "Faded away."

"Numbers faded away completely now… When all the numbers are gone from your mind, just say, 'Gone.'"

Client says, "Gone."

"Now let your mind be filled with nothingness."

Please note that it is very important that the client actually masters making the numbers disappear, and that they signal you by saying so. You want the client to be both physically and mentally relaxed, in order to be more in control of their experience. There have been cases where the client only relaxed physically with the process. While the hypnotherapist assumed that their client had dispelled all the numbers from their mind because they had stopped saying numbers, in fact the client merely stopped speaking because they relaxed so much that speaking was difficult. This is a pleasant level to go to, but it is only half of what it takes to achieve the degree of mind mastery needed for pain control. So always have them tell you when all numbers have been dispelled. Once they have accomplished this, we can apply this new skill of thinking about numbers and sending them away, to being aware of pain and then sending the pain away.

Testing Techniques
Eye Catalepsy
Eye catalepsy is a very useful hypnotic test that uses the suggestion that the client is no longer able to open their eyes. When the client experiences their subconscious responding in this physical manner, it brings an awareness of the trance state to their conscious mind. This is often a pleasing moment for the client because they now know their subconscious is actually responding, and that is why they came to a hypnotist in the first place—to get help from their subconscious creative intelligence. When their subconscious responds to the suggested behavior ("try to open your eyes and find them locking down tight") the client experiences deepening by realization.

Note that you never say that their eyes are actually glued shut. The critical faculty would immediately become engaged with such wording and object. The correct wording is "as if" they were glued. The "as if" wording is acceptable to the client's critical faculty.

Begin as follows:

> "In a moment I am going to count backwards from five down to one and you are going to experience your highly responsive subconscious mind doing it's perfect work for you. On or before the number one, your eyelids are locked down tight. Any attempt to open them causes them to lock down tighter."

Place your finger on the bridge of their nose, just between the eyebrows.

"Five… Eyelids locking down tight.

Four… Eyelids sealing shut, as if glued.

Three… Eyelids pressing down and sealing shut.

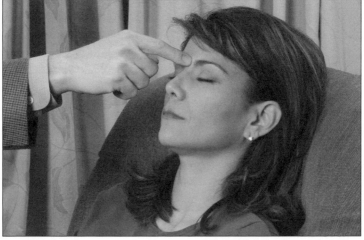

Eye Catalepsy

> Two… Any attempt to open your eyes causes them to lock down tighter."

Pull away your hand.

> "One… Try to open your eyes and find them locking down tight."

Pause a few seconds while the client attempts to open their eyes, then continue.

> "Alright, stop trying and go three times deeper into hypnosis."

Arm Catalepsy

The arm catalepsy technique is much like the eye catalepsy in principle. I usually use the eye catalepsy first before going on to larger muscles with the arm catalepsy. Remember that hypnosis is a learned skill. By the time you make use of the arm catalepsy technique, you will have guided and coached the client through numerous other inductions, deepening techniques, and testing methods. That way, when you perform the arm catalepsy, they will have developed a certain degree of hypnotic sophistication and created communion of mind and body, and of conscious and subconscious.

In the post-hypnosis debriefing, clients will often describe their experience of this test by saying, "It was like my arm wouldn't move, no matter how hard I consciously tried to bend it." That means they got a physical experience of their subconscious acting on the suggestion to create stiffness in the arm. This is an excellent stepping-stone toward succeeding with future therapeutic suggestions.

Begin as follows:

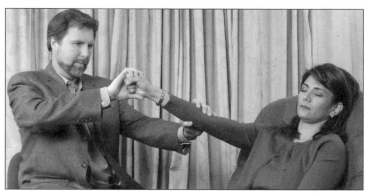
Starting position for Arm Catalepsy

"Now I'm going to show you a power you may have never been in touch with before."

Ball the client's hand into a fist and stretch out their arm so that it is straight as you say the following:

"Make a tight fist. Bring your arm up and straight."

Let go of their fist and use both hands to squeeze the wrist, elbow, and shoulder, nonverbally communicating that they should become firmly locked. Do not support the weight or position of the arm as you say the following:

"Lock your wrist, lock your elbow, lock your shoulder… That's right."

Now let go of the arm completely. The client's arm should stay locked out straight all by itself.

"Your arm is now growing powerfully stiff and rigid, just as stiff and rigid as if it were a steel bar. That's right, completely stiff and rigid through the whole length of your arm, just like a steel bar. Any attempt

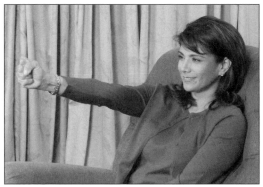
Ending position for Arm Catalepsy

to bend or lower your arm causes it to grow even more stiff and rigid now. Go ahead and try to bend or lower your arm, and find it growing even more stiff and rigid."

Give the client a few seconds to try to bend or lower their arm, then continue. As an option, you can have the client open their eyes while they try to bend their arm.

"Good, now stop trying. Now that you've developed a responsive subconscious, you'll see how truly easy it is to use the power of your mind to create the health that is your birthright. I'm going to tap you on the forehead, and when I do, your arm softens and falls limply to your side, taking you three times deeper into hypnosis."

Place one hand under the client's arm so that you can catch it when it falls and then tap them on the forehead. Catch their arm and then drop it by their side.

After reading this book in its entirety, you can make use of the Appendix, which includes examples of the induction, deepening and testing methods combined into a single script.

CHAPTER 5

Using the Right Script to Accelerate Healing

For most hypnotherapists, the question eventually arises of where to find the right scripts for each specific health issue. These days you can find all kinds of scripts that have been written for a wide variety of health issues. Some of them are well written, and some are just inappropriate and ineffective. Even if they were all well written you would not find a script for every single health issue. What happens when your next client presents a health issue for which you cannot find a script?

By learning to create your own personalized scripts, you will never have to worry about finding the right script for your client. Creating personalized scripts requires you to conduct an effective interview. By asking the right questions, you can get all the information you need to design therapeutic suggestions and healing imagery. When you get the information from the *client*, instead of a book or other source, the suggestions and imagery you create will be far more effective because they specifically address the unique needs of each individual. Generic scripts invariably either leave out something that is relevant or include something that is irrelevant to the particular situation of the person you're working with.

During your first or second session with a client, it is important to conduct an in-depth interview. The rest of this chapter is about the right questions to ask during the interview to make sure you get comprehensive information to create your personalized suggestions and imagery.

Get the Physician's Involvement
As usual, this person is under a physician's care and the physician agrees with using hypnotherapy as an adjunct to the client's care. If you are a hypnotherapist and not also a licensed health care provider, this is a good time to suggest that the client ask their physician to describe the proper function of their body, and what has to happen internally for proper function to be restored. Then proper function, as described by their physician, can be integrated into their healing suggestions. Just keep in mind that the vocabulary cannot be so technical that the client does not understand the meaning of the description. Diagrams and illustrations from the physician can be helpful visual aids.

If you are a licensed health care provider, you may already know the pathology of their disease. You can use your knowledge to program proper function. Be as specific as possible while remembering to keep your vocabulary understandable to the client.

Ask the Right Questions
In your interview, you will want to gather all the information you need to create effective healing suggestions. This will include the client's physical, mental, and emotional

condition with their issue, as well as the history of the issue, the client's actual goals, and possibly even the purpose the issue serves in the client's life.

1) Ask about the physical manifestation of the issue.

First you need to understand how the client's issue manifests itself physically. What does it feel like? What parts of the body are affected? What symptoms do they have? How long have they had them? What makes it better? What makes it worse?

By understanding how the issue manifests (the problem), you can then help the client program their subconscious with the reversal (the solution). Each undesirable aspect of their condition can then be addressed with a specific therapeutic suggestion.

As an example, imagine you're working with a 20-year old male who has asthma. In the interview, you ask about the physical manifestation of the asthma. He tells you that when he has an exacerbation, his *chest feels tight*, he starts *wheezing*, and he *feels like he can't get enough air*. He also tells you that *he tends to have more exacerbations in the spring*. He plays basketball for a city league and always *has to use his inhaler during games and occasionally can't finish a full game*. He has also noticed that the *attacks/exacerbations are worse during times of high stress*.

2) Ask about related thinking patterns.

You will want to discover the client's limiting thoughts about the issue. Understanding, and then reversing, the underlying limiting thoughts related to the health issue is a big part of the client's self-healing. We know that placebo power is the healing action of positive thought, but it's important to realize that limiting thoughts also have power—a counterproductive or "nocebo" effect. As important as it is to program positive, healthy thinking patterns, it is equally important to uncover and reverse chronic limiting thinking patterns that may otherwise stand in the way of complete healing.

The stem sentence completion process can be a very effective way to help the client get in touch with the underlying limiting thoughts related to their health issue. Here is how this works. First, tell the client that you are going to prompt them with the beginning or "stem" of a sentence. Instruct them to repeat the beginning you give them and then finish the sentence with their own ending. Here are a few examples of some stems you could use with your asthma client.

"About me and my lungs, I think..."

"About me and my health, I think..."

"My worst thought about my lungs is..."

"My worst thought about my body is..."

"My worst thought about my health is..."

You can also make use of some of their own more loaded statements as stems to check for deeper thoughts related to the issue. Say for example that the client said that he often has the thought, "There's not enough for me." You could use this as a stem very easily by having him fill in the blank. Prompt the client with the sentence, "There's not enough... X ...for me."

Have him repeat the sentence out loud and fill in the blank. In this case, your asthma client says, "*There's not enough love for me.*"

3) Ask about related emotional patterns.

Ask the client to review some recent experiences of their issue and tell you about the emotions they were feeling during these experiences. This is important information because their emotional patterns are a result of their thought patterns. These emotional patterns will, in turn, influence their thinking as well, creating a snowball effect. Negative, heavy emotions block the immune function and often act as triggers that either initiate or exacerbate health conditions.

Let us say your asthma client tells you the last exacerbation happened at his workplace. The deadline for an important project was coming up and there was still way too much to be done. He started to feel *stress* and eventually *overwhelming anxiety*. Within the hour he began wheezing and felt *disappointed in himself*. With this information, you can use the positive reversals of these emotional states linked to higher quality thoughts in the therapeutic suggestions, suggesting calmness, relaxation, feeling at ease, and being satisfied with himself. The feeling tone encouraged by the suggestions helps to open the critical faculty and anchor the new positive ideas in the subconscious.

4) Ask about when the issue started.

The body is a communication device. Looking at what was going on in the client's life when the health issue began can be very telling. Often the body is attempting to communicate or reflect our thoughts, whether they be positive and expanding, or negative and limiting. Inquire about what was going on in the client's life as far back as twelve months before the health issue began.

In this case, the client reveals that his asthma began when he was seventeen. His *parents got divorced in the spring of that year*. He moved in with Dad and only got to visit

Mom on holidays. And so we see the origin of the "there is not enough love for me" thought. In this example, it may be that the body is communicating the idea of not having enough love with the experience of not having enough air. And maybe it's not a coincidence that it is felt in the chest where love would usually be felt. If that turns out to be the case, we could suggest a behavior of self-appreciation. There is always more than enough love when we learn to appreciate ourselves, reconnect with our innate innocence, and cultivate self-forgiveness.

5) *Ask about what the client wants.*

Most people are in the habit of talking about what they don't want. "I don't want my ulcer." "I don't want cancer." "I don't want to get an asthma attack when I'm playing basketball." Talking about what is not wanted creates images of the problem and reinforces the issue. It gives nothing positive for the subconscious creative intelligence to move toward, which inhibits the healing process. Have the client tell you exactly what results they want to achieve by doing hypnotherapy. Have them be specific and speak in positive terms. This is important for a variety of reasons. By having the client tell you what they do want, in their own words, they create health-producing images and begin moving their creative intelligence in a productive direction.

Coach your client to tell you what they do want, specifically and stated in the positive. "I don't want my ulcer" becomes "I want my stomach lining to heal, becoming fully intact, and my digestive juices to regain balance." "I don't want cancer" becomes "I want my body to only produce healthy cells that function normally." And "I don't want to get an asthma attack when I'm playing basketball" becomes "I want to breathe freely and easily when I'm playing basketball."

To help the client clarify what they want, ask them to tell you how they will know when their goal has been reached. What will be different? How will they feel? What will they be able to do that they cannot do now? Getting the client to describe their desired outcome clearly and specifically in their own words allows you to use their own words and descriptions in your therapeutic suggestions and imagery. Using the client's own words and metaphors will make the suggestions and imagery more compelling for them, and therefore more effective.

Another reason why it is important to find out from the client exactly what they want for themselves is to avoid imposing your own opinions and values on the client. Hypnotherapy is ultimately a self-help method. The ethical hypnotherapist works only on what is mutually agreed to be in the client's best interest. Instead of assuming or making up what is best for the client, the client basically tells you what direction the work will take. As hypnotherapists, it is not our place to diagnose and prescribe. Our role is to help the client clarify what they want and, as long as it's in accordance with their physician's orders, help them get it.

Here is an example of how hypnotherapy is client driven. Let us say you are working with a client who has cancer. They want you to teach them how to use self-hypnosis to sleep better at night and help control some of the nausea from their chemotherapy treatments. You tell them that regaining their natural sleep pattern is fairly simple, and that their subconscious can turn down the nausea and increase their appetite so they can eat again. You add that you can also show them how to use hypnotherapy methods to talk to their body and encourage more white blood cells to destroy the cancer cells and thereby potentiate the chemotherapy and speed up their full recovery. After hearing this last bit about communicating with white blood cells, the client says, "That part sounds a little too much like science fiction. I'd rather just work on sleeping better and increasing my appetite." At this point it is best to just do the work they want to do. You will build greater rapport with them and these results might serve as stepping stones to do more advanced work later.

6) *Ask about secondary gain.*

Secondary gain, sometimes referred to as a negative payoff, is a positive benefit received indirectly through an otherwise negative behavior or situation. A secondary gain can motivate the subconscious to create or maintain an unhealthy situation to meet needs that are not being met in any other way. It is typically an unexpected benefit that results from the situation. The patterns caused by a secondary gain are usually completely subconscious. It's important to identify any secondary gain your client may be getting from their health issue so that they can use positive means to receive the same benefit. When their needs are being met through positive behavior, the negative health issue no longer has any subconscious value and the roadblocks to healing are removed.

If there is secondary gain, it does not mean something is broken. To the contrary, it means that the client's mind is working perfectly. Their subconscious creative intelligence is working to get their needs met in whatever way it can. You just need to help the client become conscious of what it is they need, and help them find healthier ways of getting it.

It is important to be tactful when asking about secondary gain to avoid creating what I call "new age guilt." I have been involved in the human potential movement for nearly thirty years now, and I have noticed that a superficial understanding of how thought is creative can end up supporting a guilt complex. Thought is creative, but that does not mean that everything we create with it was consciously intended or desired. Bluntly saying something like, "So, why did you create the cancer?" implies that they wanted to create it and that they created it on purpose, which is certainly not the case. Though the client is innocent, false implications like these can leave them feeling guilty. That is new age guilt. Our role is to inquire, with the utmost respect, as to the possibility of secondary gain resulting from the health issue, and assist the client in finding ways to get the same positive benefits in a positive and constructive manner. This will speed healing and increase their self-esteem.

Bernie Siegel, MD, author of *Love, Medicine and Miracles*, may ask his patients why they "need" their illness. In other words, what does having the health issue "set up" in their life. How does it serve them? Perhaps the health issue has built into a crisis and the client has to take a leave of absence from their work. Now they can avoid the workplace and the "dead end" prospect of staying in a job or career that they do not like. The only problem with that is that the client has to endure suffering through the illness to get the payoff.

By identifying the benefit that they are receiving indirectly through being ill, we can help them address it through more positive means, such as looking for another job or going back to school. Then there will be no more subconscious motivation to maintain the illness.

In the case of our asthma client, he tells us that he does get *more attention* and even *more physical affection from his girlfriend* when he has an asthma attack. Each time this occurs, he notices himself having the thought that *she must really care* about him. After discussing the concept of secondary gain, he decides that it is far better for his self-esteem, not to mention his health, to just assure himself that she cares simply because she is in his life. He also realizes that there is a healthier way to meet his physical needs—the best way to get a hug is to give one.

Putting It All Together
The final elements for designing the most effective accelerated healing suggestions are found in Chapter Six, which goes far deeper into the rules for writing therapeutic suggestions and designing healing imagery. For now, let us put together the proper therapeutic suggestions from the information we got during this client's pre-hypnosis interview. I will take the information and build up to the eventual desired outcome. In general, it is best to include the self-esteem building earlier in the programming because that is the foundation for self-love, and self-love powerfully assists in the healing process. At this point the induction and deepening have already been done and the client is in a deep trance.

> "As you go deeper into hypnotic relaxation, your subconscious mind is open and responsive to the following beneficial ideas. (Person's name), what you are about to hear is the truth about you.
>
> You are lovable. You see yourself as a lovable person, well deserving of all the best health in life. Because you now choose to see yourself as a lovable person, your bronchial tubes are always open and clear during springtime. Your bronchial tubes and lungs remain clear and open more and more now. Just as a red rose opens in the spring, so your bronchial tubes and lungs remain open in springtime.
>
> Every day and in every way, you are getting better and better now. Every day and in every way, your

bronchial tubes and lungs remain open and clear and because they do, you get plenty of oxygen-rich air deep into your lungs when playing sports like basketball. Your chest feels open, relaxed, and loose when you breathe. Because more oxygen-rich air is getting deep into your lungs, every day and in every way you feel physically stronger now. Because your bronchial tubes are clear and open when playing sports, you breathe freely and easily when you play basketball and easily finish each game.

(Person's name), you now gladly accept all the love that surrounds you. You more freely show appreciation to yourself and others. Your inner voice is self-assuring. Your inner voice tells you that you are important and loved. You are satisfied with yourself. You are filled with self-love now. You warmly give hugs and affection to the ones you love and you gladly receive their love in return.

Because you enjoy doing things that are good for you, you practice self-hypnosis every day. Because you practice self-hypnosis daily, life is more calming to you. More and more now, you stay centered all day. You are safe. You are strong. Your body is strong and healthy. You are more and more happy with your increasing health. You more easily cope with life and you expect the best because you realize now that there is more than enough love for everyone.

(Person's name), your bronchial tubes are clear and open now. Plenty of oxygen-rich air deeply fills your lungs all year round. Every day and in every way you are getting better and better now. (Person's name), your bronchial tubes are clear and open now. Plenty of oxygen-rich air deeply fills your lungs when exercising and playing sports.

(Person's name), all these ideas have made a permanent impression on your responsive subconscious mind. They become your everyday experience now."

Now here we have developed a comprehensive and personalized suggestion therapy program that is far more effective than the generic, cookie cutter approach to working with a unique human being. The next part of this session would be the healing imagery. Rules for designing healing imagery are given in the next chapter.

CHAPTER 6

Speaking Subconscious: Designing Therapeutic Suggestions and Healing Imagery

Think back for a moment about the lemon exercise from Chapter Two. By simply thinking about biting into a lemon, thousands of neurochemical messengers were released, and the jaws clenched and the salivary glands reacted. Early American psychologist and philosopher William James said, "The fact is that there is no sort of consciousness whatever, be it sensation, feeling, or idea, which does not directly and of itself tend to discharge into some motor effect." This idea (that every thought causes a physical reaction) is known today as the Law of Impressed Thought.

The Law of Impressed Thought
The Law of Impressed Thought states that *every impression on the mind has a physical expression.* I touched on

this briefly at the end of Chapter Two, but it deserves more emphasis because it is so important in understanding how to write effective suggestions and construct healing imagery.

Imagine you're telling a joke at a dinner party and you mess up the punch line. Feeling a little embarrassed, you start to blush. The blushing is caused by a thought. The thought that your listeners will laugh at you, instead of the joke, brings about a physical reaction—an immediate increase in blood flow to the surface of the face. That's the Law of Impressed Thought. The thought of being laughed at was impressed on the mind, and the autonomic nervous system reacted, causing a redistribution of blood flow, increased heart rate, and shallow breathing.

Just as fear of ridicule, failure, and disapproval engage the law, so does expecting approval, optimism, and love. Harvard researcher W. B. Cannon found that thoughts and feelings of love improved circulation, improved digestion, and even put a sparkle in the eyes. Therapeutic suggestions make intentional use of the Law of Impressed Thought. They are simply ideas presented in such a way that they are most likely to be expressed physically.

Thinking of the subconscious as the software and the brain and body as the hardware, realize that the hardware always does just what the software tells it to do. Suggestion therapy can be thought of as reprogramming the subconscious software to get the brain-body hardware to do something new or differently.

Getting suggestions past the conscious mind's critical faculty requires the ideas to be worded in the most effective way. There are nine general rules to keep in mind when designing effective therapeutic suggestions, but before presenting them, let's look at what the client can do with their mind to make suggestion therapy more effective.

Directing Placebo Power and the Client's Mindset

Belief mobilizes the power of the subconscious mind to block pain and release the natural healing ability of the body. The client needs to have some degree of desire, belief, and expectation before you begin the hypnosis. That's what increasing responsiveness is all about. Both Emile Coué (1857-1926) and Dave Elman thought that these attitudes were essential. Some clients will come for hypnotherapy thinking, "I'm willing to try, but I don't really think this will work." That's the wrong attitude. The right attitude says, "Yes, this will help me." That's the attitude that enables the placebo effect and taps into the power of belief.

The right attitude is created in part by how you approach the client. When someone is in pain or distress, they can easily sense your attitude. Their critical faculty is open and their subconscious can sense insecurity and doubt a mile away. If you approach the sick or injured with an attitude that says, "Let's try, but I'm not sure how well you'll do," the client will pick up on it right away and probably adopt a similar attitude. The best attitude for the sick or injured is, "Yes, teach me how to help myself." So the best attitude for you to have is, "Yes, I can absolutely teach you how to help yourself."

It is essential that you maintain an attitude of faith. Strong faith in the power of the mind to heal and relieve pain is *absolutely essential* for the practitioner of medical hypnotherapy. Some of those reading may not be in the practice of using faith as a scientific healing technique, but the research has shown that faith is a predictable agent of healing. I am not talking about religious faith, but rather a confidence that is so perceptible by others that it is contagious. When a medical hypnotherapist approaches a client with this kind of faith, it makes all the difference.

Who to Hypnotize First

This kind of confidence comes with practice, not from reading a book or watching a DVD on hypnotherapy technique. Confidence in one's ability to perform the session is best developed by just doing sessions. Seeing people release their pain and heal their bodies before your very eyes is how you develop the ultimate confidence. While you are learning, get as many volunteers as possible. Practice as often as possible. Tell people you are learning hypnosis and they will tell you that they have always wanted to try it. Perfect! Say, "I would be happy to show you how hypnosis works. How about Saturday morning?" Then hypnotize yourself that morning before meeting your friend. While in hypnosis, mentally rehearse the techniques. Each time you do, you are creating a subconscious blueprint for how to do the session. Then later, when you actually meet your friend and do the session, you'll know how to act.

Faith is simply an inner conviction that what is yet to be, *will* be. It is a catalyzing agent, and a powerful one at that. It is necessary to establish expectation as well. Expectation comes about by actually experiencing incremental accomplishments. Perhaps the client can reduce their chronic pain by 50 percent in a session. That builds the expectation that complete relief will soon be achieved. Belief and expectation develop as we get the right thoughts and images into the subconscious.

A simple way to keep everyone's attitude in the right place is to coach the client to actually say the word "yes" occasionally. Sporadically coach them to say "yes" at the beginning of a therapeutic suggestion. This will help them maintain an attitude that says, "Yes, my deeper mind does help me. Yes, I accept these positive ideas. Yes, I am healing myself now."

Nine Rules For Designing Effective Suggestions
1) State the goal in positive terms.
State what you do want, not what you do not want. The subconscious speaks in pictures and responds to imagery. The problem with negative statements is that they present an image of what we do not want. Consciously we understand the negation, but the subconscious only understands the picture. For instance, say someone is working with weight control and using the affirmation, "I no longer eat chocolate éclairs before going to bed." The subconscious mind thinks in images, and the only images here are of eating éclairs and going to bed, in that order. That means the impression being made on the mind is of eating éclairs before going to bed—precisely the behavior we do not want. Instead, one might say something like, "I now enjoy eating more fruits and vegetables every day. In the evening I feel filled with love, and my stomach feels full all night long."

If you have to state the problem, put the solution in the very next sentence. For example, when using verbal first aid to help someone who is bleeding we might say, "Stop that bleeding. Conserve your blood. Like turning off a faucet, close those blood vessels now!" Here the negative image of bleeding is followed immediately by imagery of the desired solution of closing the blood vessels.

2) Use the present tense.
Effective directions to the subconscious must present the goal occurring now. A statement like, "You are healthy" can leave the creative mind saying, "Okay, I'll be healthy later." Word your therapeutic suggestions so that the client sees themselves making the desired improvements _now._ A far more effective therapeutic suggestion would be, "Because you are learning how to relax with self-hypnosis, your resting blood pressure lowers to your goal of 130 over 80 now."

3) Paint pictures.

Use words that paint pictures. The subconscious speaks in pictures, stories, and metaphoric imagery. Like in dream imagery, we need to speak in pictures too. For the hypertensive client you could say, "Your blood pressure normalizes," but a more effective statement for the subconscious is, "Your blood vessels are more flexible now. As your healthy heart beats, it sends nutrient rich, oxygenated blood through your supple arteries and veins. Your arteries and veins expand elastically with each heartbeat. Your arteries transport healthy red blood to every part of your body. When you check your blood pressure at home, you are happy to see that the meter reads 128 over 78 and you smile."

4) Give a reason.

Suggestions are made stronger and more compelling by giving a reason why the new behavior or experience occurs. For example, you are far more likely to follow my suggestion to give a reason in your suggestions if I give you a good reason why you should do it. The hypnotic suggestion is more likely to fill the conscious mind and then be accepted by the critical faculty and passed to the subconscious when it is linked to something that seems logical.

The subconscious is constantly making associations, and is primarily interested in two types of information—meaning (A means B) and causality (B occurred because of A). Therefore, you can give the subconscious what it is looking for by using reasons in your suggestions. Reasons link ideas together in the mind. It is most effective to link something that is either observably true or under the client's control to the desired outcome, as in, "Because you exercise every day and eat healthy, nourishing foods, you recover quickly and experience renewed health and vitality now." Because exercising and eating healthy foods are under the client's control, and recovering quickly and renewed health are now linked to those behaviors, the client is now in control, albeit indirectly, of how quickly they recover and experience renewed health. That is the power of reasons.

Another way to use reasons to strengthen suggestions is to use something called an "implied causative." In an implied causative, two or more ideas are joined together in such a way that they seem to be related even though they may have little or nothing to do with each other. For example, you could say, "As you relax and go deeper into hypnosis you notice that your breathing is becoming slower, deeper, and calmer now."

5) *If it seems too great, make it incremental.*
In order for a therapeutic suggestion to be effective, it must be believable. If the goal seems too good, too big, far off, or nearly impossible, you will need to incorporate the progressive present tense. For example if you are working with someone lying in a hospital bed after a car accident, a suggestion like, "You are now healthy" is sure to be rejected by the subconscious because the statement is so clearly contradicted by the reality of the situation. Instead, an incremental suggestion like, "You are now becoming more and more comfortable with each passing hour…" is much more believable and therefore much more likely to be accepted and acted upon by the subconscious. To make your suggestions incremental, incorporate words and phrases which indicate change over a period of time, like "more and more now," "every day and in every way," "becoming," "growing," and "greater and greater."

6) *Include timing.*
Avoid words like "will," "soon," and "tomorrow." To the subconscious the only time is now, the present moment, and

tomorrow is always a day away. "Will" could mean sometime in the future, but not necessarily right now. For example, the statement, "You will be happy" could mean tomorrow, or thirty years from now when you retire. This kind of ambiguity can render ineffectual what would otherwise be a perfectly fine suggestion. Whenever possible, include specific information about when or under what circumstances the suggested behaviors and experiences take place. If something is supposed to happen on or before a specific date, use the date in your suggestions. You can also specify the relative timing of something, as in: "You are healing faster than anyone expects."

7) Suggest action, not the ability to act.
If the suggestion is that the client has the ability to heal quickly, that is exactly what they will have: the ability, not the rapid healing. Instead, suggest to the client's subconscious mind that they take action and do what they need to do to heal rapidly. Suggesting action also gets the client involved in their own healing process, which can be extremely beneficial. When suggesting action, be sure to connect taking the action with achieving the goal as in, "You exercise and stretch your lower back regularly as recommended by your physical therapist, and your back is stronger and healthier each day." By doing something that is logically associated with the goal, the main objective is achieved.

8) Use positive emotions.
Strong emotion helps to open the critical faculty so that what you are suggesting can make a more powerful impression on the subconscious. Use words that generate compelling positive images. Create positive imagery that is emotionalized. Use exciting, powerful language—words that have emotional impact and excite the imagination. Try to use one or more emotional modifiers in each sentence.

9) Be specific and keep it short.
Use language that is easy to understand. Avoid abstract concepts and generalities. For instance, if working with asthma, don't leave it at, "You breathe better." That's too general. It is more effective to say, "Because your bronchial tubes are open and clear, you breathe more easily all the time now."

How to Create Imagery that Heals
In the same way dreams are our subconscious intelligence communicating information to the conscious mind about our inner world of feeling and intuition, healing imagery is the conscious mind communicating information to the subconscious intelligence about what to heal and how to heal it. This part of a medical hypnotherapy session takes the idea of painting pictures to a deeper and more profound level.

Imagery is typically used at the end of a session. After inducing and deepening trance and delivering therapeutic suggestions, guide the client through a kind of mental movie in which they first experience themselves taking the actions which lead to their goal and then see things as they will be when the goal is achieved. The imagery will create a blueprint at the level of the subconscious—a set of instructions in the form of pictures that tell the subconscious creative intelligence what to do. Just as a student of architecture learns to draw blueprints in a way that shows the builders what to build and how to build it, the hypnotherapist must learn to use healing imagery in a way that will convey the goal to the subconscious intelligence and what has to happen for it to be achieved. When the blueprint of health is understood by the subconscious it will build a beautiful temple of health for the spirit of the client to enjoy.

Paint a Picture of What We Want

Healing imagery, just like healing suggestion, paints a picture of what we want rather than what we do not want. Researchers tell us that by the time a child is five, they have been told, "No" 40,000 times. That is a lot of programming! "No. You can't get on your mommy's new couch with your juice. You will spill your juice, and your mommy will get mad," says the babysitter. Then when the babysitter is not looking, what does the child do? Their subconscious has been told what to do. The pictured instructions were clear enough: "Get on couch, spill juice, get mommy mad." Pretty clear. So they spill the juice on the new couch and when the babysitter finds out and angrily asks, "Why did you do that?" With a puzzled look, the child says, "I don't know…" And when mommy gets home, she will ask the very same question and get the same answer. In most cases the child's response is the actual truth. They consciously do not know why they "get on couch, spill juice, get mommy mad."

Even though most of you reading were also told "No" over and over again as children, please break the habit and say what you do want. Paint pictures of the desired and proper action steps toward healing and then pictures of the healing being complete.

I remember talking with a physician once, while I was working as a paramedic, about a diabetic client he was working with. The client's blood sugar levels were so high that she was literally in a coma. He had the nursing staff start an intravenous drip of insulin to lower the blood sugar. He said that if she would just stop eating sugarcoated pastries, she would not be in this condition. Then, in a sad voice, he continued, "But she eats them every day."

In a case like this, the client's dietician might outline a specific regimen of more protein from lean meat, fish, and poultry, more vegetables, some fruits, and slow-burning complex carbohydrates like spelt bread and wild rice. The healing imagery could be as follows:

> "(Person's name), imagine that you are preparing delicious food for your evening meal. The bright green broccoli and orange carrots look so appealing to you as they steam on the stove. The seasoned fish roasting slowly in the oven crackles a little, and as you smell the delicious aroma, you think to yourself, 'This must be what it's like to be in the kitchen of a fine French chef,' and you smile to yourself…
>
> Imagine, sense, and feel that you're sitting down to eat now. When you sit down to eat, you feel proud of yourself for creating such a wonderful meal. It is very tasty and you are pleased with yourself. When you finish that plate of healing food, your stomach is full and you feel satisfied."

Paint word-pictures of the client doing the things that involve them in their own self-healing.

> "(Person's name), imagine that you are enjoying your daily walk. Imagine, sense, and feel that you're breathing in the fresh morning air as you walk in the park near your house. You smile, literally stopping to smell the roses that line the walking path. The sweet smell of the roses satisfies you."

Because many diabetics cannot eat foods loaded with white sugar or high fructose corn syrup, they often feel deprived of sweet and sugary foods. So here we suggest that they get their sweetness for the day by smelling the roses.

> "Then you start walking again, picking up the pace and thinking to yourself with each step you take that your blood sugar level is balanced all day at 110, and you are glad about that. You carry one-pound weights in each hand and swing them as you walk. You feel free and happy, so you walk for 30 minutes or more every day now. Imagine this as vividly as you can while I am quiet, (person's name.) Then when it feels complete, just nod your head."

In the above case, the physician has asked the client to exercise for 30 minutes daily as stated in the imagery. This will lower their blood sugar and help to increase their metabolism all day, making it far more likely that the desired blood sugar level of 110 will be achieved.

Include All the Senses

Although we refer to it as imagery, the content should not be limited to purely visual representations. The most effective imagery sessions include all the senses—incorporating auditory, tactile, olfactory, and even gustatory descriptions into the imagery to make the experience more vivid and real. In addition to the five physical senses, it is important to also include descriptions of the desired internal experience—the thoughts and emotional states.

In the case of a client healing from knee surgery, you could begin with some imagery of them taking some positive action that leads to their recovery. Notice how this imagery includes auditory, tactile, and emotional elements in addition to the visual content.

> "Now imagine, sense, and feel that you're working with your physical therapist. See them helping you move and bend your right leg at the knee. You feel

surprisingly comfortable, and you can flex your knee with ease and comfort. Hear your physical therapist telling you how quickly your knee is healing. You feel pleased because you can feel that your knee is stronger and more flexible now with each passing day."

Next we guide them through imagery in which they have already achieved their outcome—full and comfortable use of the right leg. The client in this example vacations in Colorado each summer where they enjoy taking day-hikes in the mountains and foothills.

"(Person's name), vividly imagine now that it is next summer, and you are on your vacation in Colorado. See yourself studying a map of a moderate day-hike that you really want to do. Now imagine, sense, and feel that you are there now and you are actually walking the mountain hiking path you planned to walk right now. You walk with comfort and ease. You can hear the occasional leaf or twig crunch under your hiking boots. The mountain air smells of pine. The sky is blue and has a few white clouds. It's a pleasant temperature for walking and every few minutes a gentle breeze cools you. Your legs feel strong and stable as they take you deeper into the forest. You're so happy to be out hiking again. You feel connected with nature. You are strong and healthy."

Associated vs. Dissociated Imagery

Associated imagery is imagery seen from the first-person perspective—seeing things as if you were actually there, looking out of your own eyes. Dissociated imagery is imagery seen from a third-person perspective—seeing yourself in the scene as if looking through the eyes of an outside observer. So in associated imagery, you are actually in the movie, and in dissociated imagery you are watching a movie with you in it.

In general, people experience a stronger physical and emotional response to associated imagery than dissociated imagery. To increase the effect of positive imagery, make it associated. Because associated imagery will seem more real, the experience will be more powerful. However, if the client has a lot of pain, you can use dissociated imagery to decrease the intensity for them. Seeing their body from a dissociated perspective will commonly reduce the pain experience.

Four Fillings Drilled without Pain

I recently had my teeth cleaned and during the exam, my dentist, Michael Davis, DDS, found three molars that had cavities. We scheduled my next visit for filling them and discussed removing all the old mercury amalgam fillings as well. Michael is one the most progressive dentists you will find and he readily agreed and even encouraged me when I suggested using my self-hypnosis methods for pain control during the drilling and filling.

The appointed day arrived. We had decided to fill the three new cavities, one of which was below the gum line, and remove one of the mercury fillings and replace it with a composite free of heavy metals—four fillings in all. Michael gave me a couple of minutes to go into self-hypnosis and achieve a level of control over the pain stimulus.

My process was to use the eye fixation induction, deepen with the Elman eye closure, then tell my body to become deeper relaxed with each passing moment. I told myself that as long as I keep my eyelids relaxed so much they won't work, I feel completely comfortable. For additional pain control, I put saliva in my mouth and said to myself that my body responds to my positive thoughts, and that the teeth of my lower jaw were all numb and completely anesthetized during the dentistry and healing period afterward.

After those autosuggestions, I started to use imagery. I imagined myself floating out of my body (dissociation) and looking down on Dr. Davis and his assistant. From there I floated out and away even further to one of my favorite vacation spots in Hawaii. My wife and I often vacation in Hawaii, and on one of our visits we found a secluded beach on the north shore of Oahu. That's where I put myself for the bulk of the drilling. I suggest you interview your pain control clients for a place they would rather be, instead of in the hospital or dentist's office. Since I had gone to a beach in my mind, I was able to integrate the drilling and suction sounds very easily. They became the pleasant sound of ocean waves and wind. To make the imagery more effective, I imagined I was walking barefoot in the warm sand. I intentionally focused on the warmth of the sand, because if my feet are warm, that keeps the parasympathetic nervous system engaged.

At one point while I was enjoying being at the beach, I thought to myself, "My jaw and teeth are filled with endorphins." I imagined a protective layer of endorphins in the nerve roots of my lower jaw and teeth. And soon I was floating—floating in bliss, thinking, "Dentistry is a great way to get an endorphin rush!" With that thought I chuckled, and Michael checked in, asking, "Is everything all right?" I gave him the thumbs up and he went back to drilling and filling—sculpting the composites like an artist shaping a marble statue.

How Long Does an Autosuggestion Last?
The above procedure took about two hours. For a procedure of that length, if I had been using chemical anesthetic, it probably would have worn off and I may have needed

a second injection. But since an autosuggestion does not wear off like a shot of lidocaine does, Dr. Davis didn't have to stop for me to re-administer the self-hypnosis. The autosuggestion operates until it is replaced by another idea. As is the standard and correct protocol, we did have the painkiller on stand-by. We prearranged that if I felt pain I would raise my right hand up to signal him to use the lidocaine. But the only sensations I perceived were the pleasure of being on the beach and, twice, the experience of a slight tingle, almost like a bit of electricity. That is all. It was quite pleasant, in part due to the fact that I did not have the epinephrine or nitrates that are commonly mixed with the painkiller.

Visual, Auditory, and Kinesthetic Imagery

Everyone represents the world and their experience of it internally in the form of sensory data, most of which is visual, auditory, and kinesthetic. Individuals tend to favor one or the other sense and come to think, remember, and imagine things primarily in terms of the sense in which they are strongest. One person may be primarily auditory and can listen to a set of instructions and be able to perform the task, while another person who is primarily visual would be better prepared if they saw the task demonstrated. And a person who is primarily kinesthetic may learn faster by just trying it.

Everybody has the ability to use all the sensory systems, but the degree of skill and ease with which they are used will vary from person to person. When designing healing imagery, keep in mind that everyone is different. One client may be primarily visual and secondarily auditory and kinesthetic. Another may be primarily kinesthetic and secondarily visual and auditory. The imagery must be described in terms most appropriate for the sensory mode of the client.

I have heard from quite literally hundreds of people who are primarily auditory or kinesthetic that, "Guided imagery doesn't work for me." That is because the guide used primarily visual language. "See the red roses as you enter the garden." If you have trouble seeing the roses and the garden, there is nothing there for you. So you have to learn how to determine which sensory system is primary for each person. That way you can adapt your script to suit each individual.

Think about a Bell Ringing

To determine how to adapt your wording to your client's primary sensory system, I suggest asking the client to take a moment, close their eyes, and "think" about a bell ringing. Notice that I did not say to "picture," "imagine," or "visualize" a bell. Those words all imply a visual representation. The script asks the client to "think about a bell ringing." That leaves it open for them to use whatever sensory type is primary for them.

After about eight to ten seconds, ask them to open their eyes and describe how they thought about the bell. Ask what they noticed first and what they noticed most when they thought about the bell. Then ask which aspect of the bell was strongest for them—the ringing sound (auditory), the picture of the bell (visual), or the feeling of vibration (kinesthetic). This should give you a good idea of what their primary sensory type is. You can then find out their secondary sensory type by asking which aspect of the bell ringing was second strongest in their awareness.

If you were to do this test with me and find out that I am primarily visual and secondarily auditory, you could design my beach imagery in this way:

> "Tim, as you imagine, sense, and feel that you're at the North Shore beach, you look out onto the water

and see the waves gently lapping onto the sand. You hear the ocean waves crash on the sand and see the sea foam bubbling. All the sights and sounds of the beach are vivid and you feel at peace."

Asthma Imagery for Primary Visual, Secondary Auditory
Let us say you are working with a seventeen-year-old female client who has asthma. (We will stay with a similar case as in the earlier chapter to build on the information presented.) She plays basketball for her high school team. She normally uses her inhaler once before a game and once or twice during the game. Her parents, physician, and coach all encourage her to keep playing, but she often worries that the asthma will become too serious and that she will have to stop. She has a high level of motivation and agrees to practice with a self-hypnosis CD twice daily. She wants to reduce her bronchospasms as well as her dependency on the inhaler. Like me, she is primarily visual and secondarily auditory. This does not mean that you cannot use kinesthetic words. Still use them, just not as often as visual and auditory words. Here is an example of the kind of imagery you would use with a client like this:

> "(Person's name), imagine, sense, and feel that you are about to begin basketball practice. As you lace up your shoes, you notice how clear your breathing is. You stand up from the bench in the locker room and go over to the mirror. Looking at yourself, you smile and take in a deep, easy breath. You see your chest rise and expand and you take in more than enough air. You exhale just as easily and you watch your chest relax naturally. You hear the exhale, and notice how clearly and openly and easily you exhale.

Now imagine that you're out on the basketball court. As you warm up, you breathe so easily and deeply. As you and your teammates practice maneuvers and plays, you hear the noise of shoes squeaking on the hardwood floor, and see your teammates running around, dribbling and making baskets. Your bronchial tubes are clear and open, your lungs are relaxed, and you can hear yourself breathing smoothly and easily."

CHAPTER 7

Important Influences on Pain Erasure and Accelerated Healing

The erasure of pain with hypnosis often seems miraculous. And from the perspective of the person in pain, it is! Pain is relative, subjective and often behavioral. Some people can sustain extreme injury and complain of very little discomfort, while others, with only a minor cut or bruise, complain of intense agony. Hypnotic pain management methods raise the pain threshold, and extend the duration of pain tolerance.

When using hypnotherapy for pain control, remember that the conscious mind can only focus on one thought at a time. So, the best way to empty the mind of the experience of pain is to fill it with pleasurable thoughts.

The Fear → Tension → Pain Cycle
The expectancy of pain causes most people to tense up in an attempt to armor or shield themselves. Unfortunately,

this response only makes the pain worse. To illustrate this, Dave Elman gives the example of someone at the doctor's office who is about to have an injection. Their expectancy of pain (which is all fear is) causes them to tense up. That makes the muscles of the arm more rigid. So now the nurse has to push harder to insert the needle properly, and that makes it hurt more.

The cycle applies universally. Think about a person with chronic low back pain who has to bend over to tie their shoes. Fearing injury, they hold their breath, tightening and guarding as they bend down. The tense muscles are then pulled on and strained a little and all of a sudden they are in pain. The moment the pain is felt, they think, "Oh no, here we go again. Standing back up is *really* going to hurt." Holding their breath again and tensing up even more, they try to stand up, further straining the back muscles. Now they're really in pain. Naturally, they worry about the pain getting worse, which creates more tension. Then that tension creates more pain, and so on. That is the fear-tension-pain cycle. The medical hypnotherapist teaches the client to stop expecting the pain, loosen the tension, and thereby reduce the pain experience.

Get in the habit of asking your clients, during the pre-hypnosis interview, what seems to trigger the pain or when they expect it to come on. Then talk to them about the fear-tension-pain cycle. Once they understand the role played by their fear and tension, explain how you will help them eliminate these first two parts of the cycle by giving them a few simple post-hypnotic suggestions (a suggestion given in hypnosis that is acted on by the subconscious after the trance is terminated) to feel calm and expect comfort in those situations where they used to tense up in expectation of pain.

It is important to remain aware of when hypnotic pain control is and isn't medically appropriate. I am not suggesting that people ignore the realistic limitations of their body. Talk to them about the difference between appropriate considerations for their bodily limitations and the unnecessary fear that just makes things worse.

After inducing trance, deepening, and testing responsiveness, you can use programming like the following to help alleviate fear and tension and break the fear-tension-pain cycle.

> "(Person's name), when doing things like bending down to tie your shoelaces, you are calm, confident, and relaxed. More and more now, your back muscles are flexible and comfortable when bending down and standing up. Because you expect to be comfortable, you are more comfortable when bending down and standing up. Your stomach muscles are stronger now and help to support your back. You are balanced and coordinated when doing things that bend and stretch your back muscles. Yes, (person's name), day by day, in every way, your spine is healing more and more now."

The example above is for a client who has had back surgery and has permission from their physician or physical therapist to do things like bending down and tying their shoes. The use of the fear reducing suggestions helps them to follow the physical therapist's recommended regimen.

Applying Placebo Power

The placebo effect is a therapeutic effect that is not directly attributable to the treatment. There are various theories about what makes placebo work. Most of them say that it has something to do with the power of positive belief. Basically, when you expect something to work, the expectation itself can bring about a positive result, like alleviation of a headache or shrinking of a malignant tumor, even if the treatment is something known to have no therapeutic properties, like a sugar pill.

Regardless of the mechanism of how placebo works, innumerable controlled studies have consistently shown that, as high as fifty-five percent of the time, people get the same therapeutic result with a placebo as with an actual treatment. Participants are of course told that they are receiving the actual treatment, even when they are not. This acts as a positive suggestion. This means that the power of positive suggestion, administered even without the catalytic benefits of formal trance, can mobilize the human body's intelligence to eliminate pain and even heal disease and injury.

Too often the placebo effect is viewed only as a statistical anomaly. Instead, hypnotherapists understand that the placebo effect proves the power of positive suggestion. Placebo is a tool to be used. Licensed medical practitioners need to learn to balance their use of positive suggestion with accurate medical information and the legal issues of informed consent.

No Nocebos Please
While most of us are familiar with the word placebo, it's lesser-known cousin, the "nocebo" is just as important to be aware of. While the word placebo comes from the Latin "placere," meaning "to please," the word nocebo comes from "nocere," meaning "to harm." A nocebo is a negative placebo—a negative, counter-therapeutic effect not directly attributable to the treatment.

Negative expectations set up by negative suggestions, nocebos, can induce illness, increase pain, and inhibit healing from injury and illness. While this word just came into use during the 1990's, hypnotherapists like Emile Coué cautioned people about the dangerous effects to their health from the "gloomy" statements of others as far back as the 1920's.

To better understand what a nocebo is, imagine a close relative of yours, for example your mother, has a life-threatening illness. You live nearby, so you often drive her to the doctor's office when she needs to go. Imagine on one of those days you have taken her there, and her doctor ran some tests and you and your mom are waiting in the examination room to hear the results. When her physician walks in, you notice a serious look and slightly pinched brow have taken the place of his usual kind expression. Today's test results show that an emergency blood transfusion is necessary. The doctor tells you to go to your local hospital right away and that he will call ahead and make all the arrangements.

When you arrive, the nurse has to start an intravenous line for the blood transfusion. Accidentally, while inserting the needle, the vein is pierced and blows up into a hematoma the size of a brazil nut. Sometimes that just cannot be avoided. The nurse bandages the wound and gets out another needle to try the other arm. As she makes her next attempt, she mutters, "Hell! Not again."

Your mom, in a bit of pain now, asks, "What's the matter?"

"This vein blew too, I'll have to try again," replies the nurse.

On her third attempt, the line is successfully established for the blood transfusion. Mom needs two pints of blood, which will take hours to slowly drip in. So you and she try to make small talk as really sick people are wheeled in for their blood. Some people are so sick, they are gray and motionless, barely able to speak with the medical staff.

After four hours in that fluorescent-lit room where people try their best to delay death, the last bag of blood is finally empty and the two of you can go soon. The nurse just has to take out the IV and bandage up Mom's arm. The nurse, being very pleasant at this point in the encounter, hands you some paperwork and tells Mom that she can go, "for now."

"For now?" Mom blurts out. "Thanks for your help, but I hope I never have to go through all this ever again."

"Oh no," the nurse says, as her expression softens and her tone turns sympathetic. "Once people get to the stage where they have to come down here for transfusions, they always have to keep coming back, dear."

Unfortunately, this is a true story—it happened in April of 2006 to my mother-in-law, Nancy, and so her daughter, of course, is my wife, Heather. Thankfully, Heather is a clinical hypnotherapist, and both she and her mom knew about nocebos. Her mom deflected it the moment the nurse uttered it, and as soon as they got away from there they both took a moment to visualize Nancy healed and happy. Nancy has not needed another transfusion.

I want to make it very clear that I am not telling this story to make the nurse wrong. She does heroic work every day that most people just could not cope with. I tell you this story because it is the quintessential setup for a nocebo. High stress and emotion, other seriously ill people who could potentially be identified with as peers, and a nurse who could be seen as an authority figure making negative forecasts, which could act like direct suggestions to Mom's subconscious creative intelligence.

Backing up to when the procedure was complete, the medical staff could have said something like, "Okay, you're ready to go now. If you have any concerns please just call the number on the paperwork I gave to your daughter. I hope you feel much better. A transfusion like this can really help."

Here's another nocebo example. While not as extreme as the last, it is common. Mr. Smith is in the hospital recovering from surgery on his shoulder. A new nurse, Mary, comes on duty in the morning and checks all her patients after being briefed by the night shift. The night shift nurse, Barney, told Mary that Mr. Smith was experiencing fairly intense pain last night and was given pain medication for it.

Mary checks on Mr. Smith, introduces herself as his nurse for the day and begins to take his vital signs. After the blood pressure cuff deflates she starts checking his wound dressing. While touching his bandages she blurts out, "How's that pain this morning? Barney, said your shoulder is still giving you some trouble."

Mr. Smith had finally gotten to sleep at 4:30 am, just a little more than two hours before the shift change. "Oh, ah, yes, I can't get comfortable, the pain is really bothering me."

Now, Mr. Smith may not say it, but he felt it. He wasn't having noticeable pain when checked by the new day shift nurse. But when she suggested pain while touching his bandages she actually strengthened the suggestion with the tactile stimulus and that's a nocebo.

We all know that it is the nurse's job to assess her patients and she wants to know if Mr. Smith needs more pain relief medication. However, in this case, she may have actually inadvertently suggested pain be perceived. Instead, Mary can say, "Mr. Smith how well are you today? Tell me about your shoulder. I want to be sure you are comfortable. Is there anything I can do to help you feel better?"

Coach your clients about the fact that some health care providers inadvertently use negative language. They aren't aware of how powerful their words are. Teach your clients to say, "Cancel, cancel." After negative suggestions are presented by other people. Then the client can say a more helpful statement that suggests a positive outcome. Mr. Smith could say to himself, "My shoulder procedure helps me move my arm with greater ease and comfort. With each passing minute my shoulder is more comfortable."

Being conscious and careful with our language choices is important for the comfort and healing of our clients, as well as for our own personal well-being.

CHAPTER 8

Overcoming the Roadblocks to Healing and Pain Relief

What if your client is doing everything their medical team is advising and they still are not healing, or they still have quite a bit of pain from their injury or illness? While they consciously want to feel better, there may be an opposing idea or influence at work at the subconscious level. This chapter will describe some of those roadblocks and how to clear them out of the way.

Your Subconscious Mind Hears Everything You Say
The subconscious is the seat of belief. What we believe creates our expectations. And what is expected has a powerful tendency to occur. This we refer to as the Law of Expectation. What your clients say out loud helps to form their beliefs and engages the Law of Expectation.

As explained in Chapter One, in order for an idea to become a subconsciously held belief, it must first get past the critical faculty. There are five primary ways to bypass the critical faculty:

- repetition
- emotion
- authority
- identification
- hypnosis

We use all five when we speak.

First, because our thoughts about our lives are mostly the same from one day to the next, we repeat ourselves a lot. We complain about the same things, tell the same stories, espouse the same points of view, and so on. So there we have *repetition*.

Second, in order to sound congruent when we talk to others we must have emotion to match what we say. So when we talk about things in either a very positive way or very negative way, we tend to generate strong *emotion* to back it up.

Third, we are each ultimately our own highest *authority*. So much so that we don't even question our own authority most of the time. If we think something and believe it enough to say it, we have already accepted it as truth.

Fourth, each of us holds an image of ourselves as we would like to be, and the subconscious is always working to close the gap between that image and the reality of who we are now. We have integrity to the degree that our self-image matches the reality of who we are. The subconscious drive toward integrity constitutes *identification* with our own self-image, which is every bit as strong as identification with an external person or group.

And fifth, when we speak without being conscious of what we are saying and how we are saying it, our speech becomes *hypnotic* because we are uncritical of it. Everything we say, be it intentional or unintentional, acts as autosuggestion. Everything we say goes out our mouth and straight back into our ears, and our subconscious hears every word.

Coach your clients to examine their habitual language. You want them to harness the power of autosuggestion to support their healing instead of hindering it. The first step is teaching them self-hypnosis and the use of intentional autosuggestion. Intentional autosuggestion is the deliberate repetition of carefully constructed statements that affirm the desired outcome and instruct the subconscious in how to achieve it.

Self-hypnosis and intentional autosuggestion shift the way the client thinks about their condition at the subconscious level, but if they are in the habit of speaking about their condition in negative terms the rest of the time, they will be counteracting their own efforts.

When someone is sick or injured, they are often asked over and over by friends and family how they are doing. Coach your clients to answer questions like these in realistic yet positive terms, to avoid complaining and commiserating, and to think and speak in terms of how they *want* to be doing and the *progress* they are making in that direction.

In addition to becoming conscious of their own speech, coach clients to become aware of what others say around them. This is part of managing suggestibility. If others are speaking in negative, pessimistic terms regarding their health issue, and the client agrees with them or even just nods or acquiesces, they are opening their critical faculty to the negative suggestions. Instead, coach your clients to be aware of what others are saying, and to politely correct them if it does not match the way they choose to think about it. By coaching their friends and family in the correct way to speak about their condition, they are also reinforcing their own positive outlook.

Organ Language

There are countless expressions in the English language that use body metaphors to describe negative states like frustration, fatigue, betrayal, stress, fear, and sadness. These kinds of expressions are known as organ language, because they frequently refer to a specific part of the body. For example, it's common to hear people speak of having a "broken heart" or complain that something is a "pain in the neck."

These statements can also act as unintentional autosuggestion and in some cases the subconscious mind will actually begin to create the condition being used in the metaphor. A member of our staff had a very concrete experience of this before she trained in hypnotherapy. A number of years ago she found herself working at a job that was out of alignment with who she was as a person and the relationship she was in at the time was also beginning to fall apart. As the overwhelm of these two situations was mounting, she kept saying to herself, "I need a break!" Not realizing what a statement like that could create, she repeated it over and over again. After few weeks of this, she broke her hand. Later she was able to look back and see how her subconscious responded to her repeated suggestion. Now she says that the experience was a gift that taught her the power of language and how we all need to learn to speak consciously.

Coach your clients to become aware of their use of organ language. Is their job killing them? Are their children giving them an ulcer? Maybe. Or maybe it's just their subconscious creative intelligence responding perfectly to their clear instructions.

Killer Stress

One of the effects of stress is that it suppresses the parasympathetic nervous system functions. This means that the immune, digestive, and reproductive systems are running on less energy than is needed for optimal health. During periods of high stress, blood flow is diverted away from these vital systems and the body's ability to maintain health is impaired. Deep sleep, which is particularly important for creating and maintaining optimal health, also becomes difficult because of the increased levels of stress hormones brought about by acute or chronic stress.

Stress occurs as a response to any type of demand. While we tend to associate stress with difficult or painful life events, stress also occurs when good things happen. Have you ever gone on vacation to enjoy some rest and relaxation only to come home just as tired as when you left? I know I have. What is so tiring about relaxing on the beach in Hawaii or going on a cruise? Nothing really, but the complete change of routine places demands on us both physically and mentally. Knowing this, I usually schedule a couple of extra days off after arriving home to rest up from resting up.

Big changes in our lives can be very demanding and can have a major impact on health if not dealt with proactively. The death of a loved one, the loss of a job, a divorce—these sort of events can be very stressful and drain the body of the vital energy needed to combat disease and maintain health. It is very common for a health crisis to manifest within twelve to thirty-six months following a period of high stress and distress.

Killer Stress and Self-Esteem
One of the underlying causes of killer stress is low self-esteem. People with low self-esteem tend to perceive themselves as being less capable of dealing with life situations. Negative beliefs about themselves and their own capabilities make these people perceive life events as being more difficult and stressful than they would otherwise seem.

Self-esteem is governed by self-thoughts—the thoughts that we hold at the subconscious level about who we are and what we're capable of. Self-thoughts color the subconscious lens through which we see ourselves and the world. For example, if a person holds the self-thought, "I am weak," they will tend to perceive life situations as being too difficult for them. For them, life is chronically demanding, so they tend to experience chronic stress. A person who holds the belief that they are weak will experience greater difficulty in handling their health issues than someone who believes that they are strong and capable.

To raise self-esteem it is important to uncover and reverse limiting self-thoughts. Reversing negative and limiting self-thoughts is what my long time friend Sondra Ray, author of *Loving Relationships Volumes 1 & 2* and *Healing and Holiness*, calls programming the truth about you. Programming the truth about you means integrating therapeutic suggestions into your self-hypnosis practice that reverse your most negative self-thoughts.

When programming the truth about you, it is not necessary to invert every single limiting self-thought. There is a hierarchy to self-thoughts. Self-thoughts about capabilities and situations rest on the foundation of deeper self-thoughts about our identity and character. Attempting to change higher-level limiting thoughts without reversing the foundational beliefs on which they are based is extremely difficult. By inverting negative self-thoughts at the level of identity and character, the higher-level limiting thoughts that depend on them lose their foundation and become easy to change.

Use the stem sentence completion process explained in Chapter Five to uncover the client's most negative thoughts about themselves and their health. You can then program the positive reversals in your hypnotherapy sessions with them as well as have the client program themselves with the truth about them as part of their daily self-hypnosis practice.

When reversing negative self-thoughts, keep the positive inversion close to the limiting idea. For example, a client says, "I'm too weak. I can't handle this cancer." The positive reversal must address both the identity self-thought ("I'm too weak") and the higher-level capability self-thought ("I can't handle this cancer"), in that order. The positive reversal for this client could be something like the following.

> **"More and more now, I see myself as a strong and capable person. Because I choose to see myself as strong and capable, I find it easier and easier to do the things I need to do to take care of myself and heal. I respond well to all treatments and medical procedures and my resourceful creative intelligence finds powerful ways to help me heal completely. I am strong."**

Adding personalized therapeutic suggestions that invert limiting self-thoughts to your client's hypnotherapy regimen will not only boost their self-esteem and reduce stress, it will also empower them to better comply with their physician's treatment strategy.

Killer Stress Can Be a Conditioned Response

Our reaction to stress-producing demands can become a conditioned response. For example, when I was working as a paramedic and my beeper would go off, I would immediately get a rush of adrenaline. I had come to associate the stress and demand of handling a medical emergency with the sound of my beeper going off.

The subconscious survival mechanism makes strong associations whenever we experience high stress. Anything that is unique or that occurs consistently in stressful situations will become associated with those situations. After the association is formed, those stimuli will trigger a stress response even if they occur in a completely different context. To this day, almost twenty years after retiring as a paramedic, I still get a small rush of adrenaline every time an ambulance blazes by with its lights flashing and siren blaring.

Discuss this with your clients and find out what stress triggers they are conditioned to. Once you've identified a trigger, you can reverse the conditioning. To do this, begin by helping the client go into a deep state of hypnotic relaxation. Then have them imagine themselves being transported to a relaxing place of comfort and peaceful ease. Help them to fill in the details of the experience so that they get the good feelings of actually being there. When the client is totally associated into the experience and is feeling good, have them imagine the old stress situations evaporating away. Instead, they imagine themselves having these relaxing, peaceful feelings during those times that used to trigger stress. This will reprogram their nervous system to respond with feelings of relaxation and calmness instead of stress.

Illness and Pain as Connection with a Loved One
We all naturally seek connection. It is one of our deeper needs, and we all desire to feel connected to the people in our lives that we look up to and love. One of the ways that people create a feeling of connection is by emulating certain characteristics of the person they wish to feel connected to. This is called "identification with a central figure," and it usually happens subconsciously.

Occasionally, in order to create a feeling of connection, people will subconsciously emulate negative traits, including illness and pain. If a favorite grandparent had migraine headaches for example, a person may develop migraines as a subconscious means of identifying with the grandparent.

The subconscious creation of real migraine headaches is a way to be like the central figure, and being like them is a way to create connection. This is an example of secondary gain. While the migraines are painful and clearly unwanted, they do provide the client with a positive benefit—a feeling of connection.

In cases like this, have your client identify other traits or characteristics of the central figure that were positive or constructive. For instance, if the grandparent was always very patient with them, the client could focus on developing their own patience with themselves and others. The key is for the client to become consciously aware of the desire for connection, and then to intentionally fulfill that desire in a healthy way by identifying and emulating positive aspects of the person. When that happens, the illness and pain have no more positive value, so the subconscious can stop creating them and create health instead.

The Suffering Meme

A "meme" is a unit of cultural information, such as a cultural practice, idea, or concept that is transmitted, verbally or by repeated action, from one mind to another. Examples of memes include political views, social customs, and religious beliefs. Part of our cultural heritage is the meme that "suffering has value."

The suffering meme says that through suffering one can absolve oneself of guilt, pay for sins or mistakes, become worthy of good things, purify the mind, or connect with a spiritual being or source. This idea has been around for so long and is so pervasive that it has become a part of our collective unconscious. Whether they are aware of it or not, many people operate on this subconscious belief. And even for those who don't, it is likely that some of the people who are close to them do.

There is no value in suffering other than the value that we mistakenly attach to it. And there is no outcome achievable through suffering that cannot be more easily, quickly, and comfortably achieved without it. In *A Course in Miracles* it states that suffering ends when the one suffering no longer values suffering.

The best way to help a client realize and accept that there is no value in suffering is to help them have a direct experience of whatever it is they expected to gain by suffering. Redirect the subconscious creative intelligence straight to the outcome. Be it spiritual connection, a return to innocence, or feeling worthy of God's love, whatever the client is seeking can be experienced directly, now. The skillful use of hypnotherapy techniques makes this possible. Any experience the mind can imagine, the mind has the power to create.

The direct experience of the desired spiritual outcome re-educates the subconscious mind, teaching it that the way to peace and spiritual connection is through positive behaviors such as forgiving, accepting, and being generous with oneself and others. Mistakes can be seen as valuable feedback and opportunities for growth instead of sins to be paid for through suffering. Mistakes teach us to improve our thinking and take a better course of action.

When people see it as more valuable to improve their quality of thoughts, emotions, and actions, and less valuable to suffer, they just heal better.

Forgiveness as a Healing Agent
Many people have forgiven their way to restored health. Resentments and grudges are toxic to the body and mind, regardless of how justified they may seem. Forgiveness frees the forgiver. It is the great liberator. It liberates you from believing that you can do nothing about the wrongs, real

or imagined that have been done to you. It also liberates your body from carrying around negative thoughts and feelings that can destroy your health over time.

Forgiveness means to make it as if that which is forgiven had never occurred. When real forgiveness is achieved, the feeling is that there is nothing to forgive. Forgiveness does not condone destructive action, nor does it invite future attack, because real forgiveness occurs as a result of spiritual growth and learning, not ignorance and avoidance. Forgiveness is a choice to free yourself from anger and hatred and let your mind, body, and spirit return to their natural state of peace, health, and serenity.

Forgive your body. Forgive your parents. Forgive your siblings. Forgive your ex-mate. Forgive your children. Forgive the government. Forgive the church. Forgive your school teachers. Forgive yourself for ever believing you needed to hold resentments to protect yourself. Resentment creates a psychological separation. But it is a separation that you have made, not a true separation. What you have made, you can unmake, and forgiveness is the way to do it.

Pain Happens—Suffering Is Optional

Pain happens. It is the body's way of telling us that something needs to be addressed. If someone trips and twists their ankle, it hurts. The pain is a feedback system telling the person to stop walking and inspect the ankle. The pain is saying, "There is an injury. You need to stop putting weight on this ankle for a few days so that it can heal." So pain is important feedback for our health. It is when we resist the pain signal or the message it is giving us that we experience suffering.

Suffering is the emotional pain caused by resistance to what is. Resistance to the situation can cause suffering when not enough proactive steps are being taken. I seldom see a person suffering who is actively doing something about their injury or illness. If the client is suffering, it may be a sign that they are in resistance to what is or that they are not taking the necessary action to handle the injury or illness. Suffering is a signal to balance accepting what cannot be changed with taking action on what can be changed.

CHAPTER 9

Dim It Down

Because each client has different needs and will respond to different styles, this book is designed to present the foundational principles so you can creatively combine methods and techniques. Understanding the underlying principles of pain control through hypnotherapy puts you in a much better position to help others reduce their suffering than if you were simply reading scripts to clients. For this reason, the following four chapters present some of the best methods for hypnotic pain control and the principles on which they are based.

Pain Reduction by Diminution

Diminution, or dimming the pain down, is one of the most effective hypnotic pain reduction methods. Diminution works through *conscious realization of control over bodily sensations*. In this method, we first guide the client through making the pain worse before sending it away. While this seems counterintuitive at first, it serves an essential purpose. To merely say to a person in pain that they can control and even erase their pain just by thinking about it will not be sufficient for most people. They will think, "Who is this quack? I've been wishing the pain wasn't there all along!" The fact that the client has been wishing and wanting the pain to vanish and that all of their wishing and wanting has been ineffective is very important. From the perspective of subconscious programming, they may be running a script that says, "When I wish or want pain to go away, pain gets worse." If that is the case, you must bypass that negative programming so that the client can respond to the diminution method—and giving the client a direct experience is the most effective way to do that. As Gil Boyne says, "Don't try to talk them into it, show them they can do it."

Because the idea of intentionally making the pain worse is so absurd, chances are good that the client has never even considered it. And if they have never considered it, then they will not have a belief that it is impossible. Because there is no opposing idea to prevent them from doing it, most people are able to make their pain worse fairly easily. And if they can make their pain worse, that means they are in control of it and can, therefore, reduce it and maybe eliminate it entirely.

After doing an in-depth interview, induce trance and have the client imagine themselves in front of a control panel that influences all their bodily functions and sensations. Then have them locate the dial that indicates their current pain level. (I use a dial in the examples in this chapter, but any kind of adjustable control will do.) When they locate the dial, have them tell you to what number it is currently set. Then tell them to turn it up. That's right, you want them to make the number higher and the pain worse. To assist them in making the pain worse, feed back some of their descriptions of the pain that you got during the interview. If they said it was a sharp, stabbing pain, say,

"By pushing the dial up to the next number, the sharp, stabbing sensation becomes more intense and the pain gets worse!" By making the pain worse, the client will realize and experience for themselves that they really are in control of their pain.

Work with a scale of zero to ten, where zero is no pain at all and ten is the worst pain they can imagine. Whatever kind of control they have on their control panel, it should be something that can be adjusted between zero and ten. Ask the client to rate their pain on this scale. If they say, for example, that the pain is currently at five, then when they are in trance and you have guided them to imagine the control dial, it will read a five, and they will be pushing it up to six as the convincer that they are in charge of their pain.

Once the client is convinced that they can control the pain, they can begin turning the dial down to reduce it. Have them do this slowly, one number at a time, and as they turn the dial down, you can help with suggestions of relaxation and comfort.

Pain Erasure with the Mind's Master Controls

This method was adapted from the diminution principle of pain elimination. First, have the client build a special place in their imagination where all bodily functions and experiences can be adjusted. People I have worked with have created anything from a special workshop, a sacred temple, or an outpost in the forest, to a space-age cockpit-like control room or a simple panel of circuits, levers, and dials. Whatever they create, it is essential that they understand that their body's functions and experiences are affected by the work they accomplish in this place.

Before inducing trance, talk a little about what type of place they would like to create. What type of architecture would they enjoy? What kind of setting and embellishments would they want? In addition to the control room, which is essential for this method of pain control, the client can create other spaces like a library of knowledge, a healing chamber, a self-hypnosis programming chamber with a movie screen for guided imagery, a healing garden for resting and rejuvenating the body, and so on. Have fun with it and remember that it is important for the client to play a creative role in designing a healing place that is right for them.

In the control room, make sure there is a dial or other control that can be adjusted to increase or decrease the pain experience, and a control to release endorphins to increase comfort and bring a feeling of joy. Other additions may be appropriate depending on the specific situation you're working with. For example, I have worked with people who had alopecia, a condition which causes hair loss that usually leaves bald patches on the scalp. They created a dial that increased the rate of hair growth on their scalp when they turned it up.

The adjustments made to these imaginary controls are translated directly into physical changes in the body. In the pre-talk, be sure to explain the Law of Impressed Thought (from Chapter Five), which states that every impression on the mind gets its physical expression. This will be familiar to your client from the lemon exercise for increasing responsiveness, where the impression made on the mind by imagining biting into a lemon had a physical expression of increased salivation and involuntary clenching of the jaw muscles.

After trance induction, deepening, and testing, guide the client to their special place and have them imagine entering the master control room where all of their bodily functions and sensations can be controlled. In the following example, the client had surgery for a fractured femur and is experiencing severe pain in the leg. As usual, this person is under a physician's care and has permission to use hypnosis to reduce their pain. Begin by speaking the following script in a slow and calming tone of voice.

> "Now imagine a beautiful passage that takes you to a special doorway. I will now count backwards from five down to the number one. When I reach the number one, be at the doorway.
>
> Five… imagine, sense, and feel yourself drifting and floating into the passage.
>
> Four… going down deeper and deeper into relaxation with each number.
>
> Three… because you imagine yourself safely floating through the passage, you go deeper and deeper into this pleasant state of hypnotic relaxation.
>
> Two… almost there now and you're feeling deeply relaxed.
>
> Number one… be at the special doorway now. On the other side of the door is a very important place. It is your special healing place.
>
> Go ahead and open the door and step through. As you step through the doorway, you are transported to the location of your special place of healing."

Guide the client through creating their special place, including the control room, healing chamber, and any other rooms, embellishments, or features they might wish to include. When they are finished constructing everything, continue.

> "Now take a few moments to fill in all the details for yourself. Make it as vivid and real as you can and nod your head when you're done."

Wait until they nod their head, then continue.

> "Good, now go to the control room for all your body's functions, sensations, and experiences and nod your head when you're there."

Wait until they nod their head, then continue.

> "You will notice a very comfortable chair here for you to sit in. Go sit in the chair. In front of it is a control panel that is all lit up, with dials, and levers. There, in front of you is the dial that controls pain sensations in your leg. The dial goes from zero to ten. If the dial read zero you would feel perfectly comfortable, and ten would be the worst pain you could imagine. Since you have been having some discomfort today, what does the dial read?"

Client says, "Six."

> "Alright, I want to show you how powerful your mind is. For only a moment, I want you to push the dial up to seven. Push it up and feel that stabbing pain intensify. Go ahead now and push the dial up to seven. When you have done that, let me know by saying the number seven out loud."

Client says, "Seven."

"Alright, now you know how powerful your mind really is. Now lower the dial back down to six. Just take a deep breath in, and as you let it out, lower the dial. When you have done that, let me know by saying the number six out loud."

Client says, "Six."

"Good, (person's name). Because you can make the pain worse, you can now use that same power to send it away. I want you to lower the dial down to the number five and notice how your leg feels more comfortable now. Just a dull ache now as you lower the dial down to five. When you reach the number five, notice yourself relaxing even more and say the number five out loud."

Client says, "Five"

Continue to guide the client through lowering the numbers on the dial while you deliver soothing, relaxing words of comfort. After reaching zero, it can be helpful to guide them to the healing chamber of their healing place to correct whatever was causing the pain.

"Now float to the healing chamber. Imagine a healing light coming in and shining on your leg. This makes any adjustments needed so that your leg heals faster and stays more comfortable. Imagine this now while I'm quiet. When you have received all the healing energy you need, nod your head."

Wait until the client nods their head, then continue.

"Good. Now you're going to leave your healing place and bring these good feelings with you. You can return here any time you would like."

At this point you would finish with specific therapeutic suggestions to quicken their recovery, boost their immune system, and help them feel more comfortable throughout their healing and rehabilitation period, and then dehypnotize.

CHAPTER

10

Dilution Is the Solution

The dilution method helps to alleviate pain of any severity. The principle at work in this method is that *you get what you focus on.* In the dilution method, ask the client to give sensory representations to their pain and also to the feelings of comfort with which they will replace the pain. Both the pain and the comfort will be represented metaphorically by a color, a sound, and a feeling chosen by the client. This gives the client a way to focus on the sensations of pain and comfort or pleasure and create those experiences in the body. Once the client can create comfort and pleasure in the body, we guide them through a process of first diluting and then flooding the painful area of their body with these good feelings, thereby eliminating the pain and replacing it with comfort.

Before formally inducing trance, have your client close their eyes and make contact with their pain by representing it with a color, a sound, and a sensation. Typically, a person in pain will choose a color like red, gray, brown or black. The sound is often described as cacophonous, blaring, siren-like, etc. And the sensation is often sharp, aching, burning, pinching, etc. Next, ask your client to disconnect from the color, sound, and feeling of the pain, and open their eyes. Let them know you are going to show them a simple way to dilute the pain and make it disappear.

After inducing hypnosis, deepening, and testing, direct the client to go to a part of their body that feels comfortable and assign a color, sound, and feeling to this portion of the body. People tend to choose shades of blue, pink, green, gold, or white to represent feelings of comfort. Sounds range from a gentle breeze in pine trees to a serene silence. And feeling descriptions include warmth, comfort, and looseness.

For the following example, imagine you're working with a client who has chronic stress headaches and has been sent to you by their physician, for medical hypnotherapy. When you ask them to close their eyes and give sensory representations to the pain in their head, they tell you that it looks red, sounds like a mallet banging against iron, and feels hot. In this example script, the parts that will change depending on the client are in parentheses. After inducing hypnosis, deepening, and testing, you would continue as follows:

> **"Alright (person's name), take your mind into your body and focus your attention on a part of your body that feels really good and really comfortable. When you're there, let me know by saying the part of the body that feels good."**

Pause while the client locates and connects with a part of the body that feels good. This usually takes about five to ten seconds.

Client says, "My arms."

> **"Give the comfort in (your arms) a color now, and when you have done that, let me know the color."**

Client says, "Blue."

> "Good. The comfortable color is (blue). Now give the good feeling in (your arms) a sound. Tune in and hear the sound that is the comfort. When you have done that, describe the sound to me."

Client says, "It's like the sound of wind moving through the trees, like a cool breeze."

> "Good. The comfortable feeling sounds (like a cool breeze). Now give the good feeling in (your arms) a physical sensation. When you have done that, describe the sensation to me."

Client says, "My arms feel like they are floating."

Now that you have these three senses involved, you can direct the client to begin moving the visual, auditory, and kinesthetic representations of comfort closer to the head where the pain is.

> "Good. The physical sensation of the comfort in (your arms) is (like floating). Now (person's name), by moving this (blue, cool breeze, floating sensation up toward your head), you can begin to feel much, much better. So begin moving that comfortable (blue) color, the sound of (a cool breeze), and the (floating) feeling (from your arms up toward your head) now. Expand the color, turn up the sound, and move the sensation (up your arms)… (and into your neck)… (and into the base of the skull). And when you have done that, just nod your head."

Wait for the client to nod their head and then continue.

> "Now imagine, sense, and feel that the pleasant (blue) color is easily moving (up to the base of your skull). Just let the (blue), comfortable color spread all the way to (the base of your skull) and notice how good that begins to feel."

Pause a few seconds.

> "Now move the pleasant sound of (a cool breeze up to the base of your skull), automatically you feel more and more comfortable."

Pause a few seconds.

> "And now move the sensation of (floating up to the base of your skull)."

Pause a few seconds.

> "(Person's name), by moving the comfortable (blue, cool breeze, floating sensation) to (the base of your skull), you are already beginning to feel more comfortable now."

Now that the color, sound, and sensation of comfort have reached the base of the skull, you can begin diluting the old pain representations with comfortable ones. Suggest that the client will feel better and better as more and more of the pleasant color, sound, and sensation replace the painful color, sound, and sensation.

> "(Person's name), you're feeling more and more comfortable now as you focus more on these good sensations, and you can feel even better now. (Your head)

is now beginning to fill with the comfortable (blue, cool breeze, floating sensation). I want you to move more (blue, cool breeze, floating sensation) into your (head) now. Just let it begin to spread all throughout your (head), diluting and washing out that (red, hammering, hot feeling) and replacing it with comfort. Wash it out by flooding the whole area with that (blue, cool breeze, floating sensation)."

Pause while the client moves the comfort throughout their head.

"As you continue making that (blue, cool breeze, floating sensation) spread throughout your (head), you notice the comfortable feeling pleasantly increasing and diluting the old, uncomfortable feeling."

Pause to give the client some time to do this.

"Move more and more of the pleasant (blue, cool breeze, floating feeling) into your (head) and you now feel better and better. Replacing the (red) with more and more of the pleasant (blue, cool breeze, floating feeling). Feeling better with each passing moment now."

Pause for about 10-15 seconds.

"Nod when you have filled your (head) with the pleasant (blue) color, the sound of (a cool breeze), and the comfortable (floating sensation). Notice that the other sensation you were feeling before has vanished, and that you are feeling better and better with each passing moment now."

Pause and wait for the nod.

> "Good (person's name), you are doing a great job. Now completely fill your (head) with the pleasant (blue, cool breeze, floating feeling) and notice that you feel completely comfortable in every way. The pleasant (blue, cool breeze, floating feeling) has completely diluted the old color and sound and you feel good! Notice how comfortable you feel and nod your head."

After the client nods their head, give them a moment to rest in comfort. Then terminate the trance with suggestions that the comfort they are now experiencing will continue, and that the original cause of their pain is being addressed by their subconscious creative intelligence.

> "(Person's name), every day, in every way, you are getting better and better. Because you practice self-hypnosis daily, you remain more calm and relaxed throughout the day. Your creative intelligence is making all the healthy changes in your body so that (your head feels comfortable and clear) more and more now. In a moment I will count from one up to the number five. When I reach the number five, you will open your eyes, feeling perfect in every way.
>
> One... A pleasant (blue, cool breeze, comfortable feeling) stays with you all day now.
>
> Two... Coming back to the room now and bringing yourself out of hypnosis completely.
>
> Three... Feeling rested and relaxed in every way.

Four... Every muscle in your body is relaxed and feeling comfortable. On the next number, you will open your eyes, feeling perfect in every way and bringing this wonderful feeling of comfort with you.

Number five... Notice how nice you feel as you open your eyes now."

Some Effective Modifications of the Dilution Method

The script above assumes that some part of the client's body feels comfortable, but that may not always be the case. You can work with generalized pain by asking the client to imagine a comfortable color, sound, and feeling representation that is outside of themselves that they can then move into themselves.

If the client has difficulty getting the full dilution, you can modify the technique by having the pain color, sound, and sensation drain out of imaginary faucets at the ends of the fingers of the hand that is on the side of the body where the pain is. If the pain is in the abdomen or lower in the body, have the pain representations drain out of imaginary faucets at the ends of the toes of the foot that is on the same side as the pain.

Either way, once the pain representations have drained out of the body, have the client imagine rinsing the pleasant representations through the faucets. Then have them imagine closing the faucets as they continue to saturate the body part or region that had pain with all the pleasant visual, auditory, and kinesthetic signals while you suggest that this creates complete comfort.

CHAPTER

11

Laying-On of Hands

In this chapter you will learn a technique known as glove anesthesia, which is one of the most common hypnotic pain erasure methods used today. In the glove anesthesia technique, we make use of direct suggestion and subconscious associations to create numbness in one of the client's hands. Once they have achieved numbness in one hand, we then suggest that they can easily transfer that numbness to the parts of the body that are in need of pain relief, just by touching them with the numb hand.

Everyone has had the experience of numbness in some part of their body at some point in their lives, be it from cold, lack of circulation to a limb while sitting or sleeping, or chemo-anesthesia. These *memories of numbness are subconscious resources.* The subconscious associates the idea of numbness with the memories of the actual physical sensations that were experienced. In the glove anesthesia technique we make use of these associations to help the client achieve pain control.

By teaching clients the glove anesthesia technique, you are helping them take a remembered experience, a subconscious resource, and bring it into their present consciousness where they can master it and turn it into a skill. We are teaching the client to take resources that they've had inside them all along and apply those resources in new ways to create the experiences they want. This general principle is very valuable in hypnotherapy work. People have all the resources they need inside them already. It's our job to help them realize this and empower them to use those resources in ways that create health and well-being.

Anesthesia vs. Analgesia
For decades this technique has been referred to as glove *anesthesia*, even though, for many people, the technique more accurately produces *analgesia*, meaning they still have sensation but they do not feel pain. This is not a failure. In fact, in some cases analgesia is actually preferable to anesthesia. For example, if the client is learning hypnosis for childbirth preparation, they may want to be able to feel the contractions as muscular waves instead of painful jabbing cramps.

Ability to achieve full anesthesia is largely a matter of practice and is directly related to the ability to achieve a deep trance. For clients who initially achieve only analgesia but wish to achieve full anesthesia, practice with self-hypnosis will help.

We recently had a person enroll in the professional hypnotherapy certification training at the Academy who had never been hypnotized. Because she had no experience with hypnosis, she was concerned that she would not be able to go into a deep trance.

In the very first week she began using the self-hypnosis process we taught her. She practiced every day, twice a day. By the third week I confirmed she was achieving deep trance. By the time we got to the healing and pain management module, she could put herself into a profoundly deep trance state.

During this module, our trainers demonstrate the power of the methods by having a clamp applied to a sensitive area of skin and a needle put through the top of their hand while using hypnosis to eliminate the pain. After we have taught the students pain control techniques, the students are given the option of trying the clamp and needle tests for themselves. Can you guess who volunteered first?

After she entered a deep trance, Robert Sapien, MD, applied the clamp to her skin. No reaction. Next, he put a needle through the top of her hand. Still no reaction. After terminating the trance, she reported that she did not feel a thing. She had perfect anesthesia! Her practice paid off and her self-esteem skyrocketed. She had mastered her mind, and by doing so, she knew that for the rest of her life she could do whatever she put her mind to.

Basic Glove Anesthesia
There are many ways to create the initial numbness in the hand needed for the glove anesthesia technique. In the most basic version of this technique, you simply suggest that the hand becomes more and more numb as you stroke it several times. Once they have achieved numbness in one hand, you then suggest that they can easily transfer this numbness to other parts of the body that are in need of pain relief by touching those areas with the numb hand. After inducing hypnosis, deepening, and testing, begin as follows.

> "Here in this hypnotic state, your subconscious mind is highly responsive to your thoughts. Because of this, you are about to experience its power to help you feel better. In a moment, I will begin stroking your hand lightly. As I do, think about your hand beginning to tingle and then becoming numb. As I continue to

stroke your hand, the tingling turns into numbness. I will stroke your hand five times, and each time I do, your hand becomes more and more numb. By the fifth stroke, your hand has lost all sensation and is completely numb."

Now stroke one of their hands five times as you say the following. Be sure to leave enough time between strokes to allow the client's subconscious to carry out the suggestions for creating numbness.

"One... Your hand is beginning to tingle as it begins to grow numb now.

Two... Your hand is becoming numb and wooden-like.

Three... Losing all sensation now as your hand grows more and more numb.

Four... It's as if it's not even there, it's so numb.

Five... Your hand is completely numb now."

Now give the client a few minutes to fully create the experience as you occasionally repeat suggestions for numbing the hand. Once the hand is numb, you can move on to transferring the numbness to the part of the body in need of pain control. In the script below, the client has had oral surgery and their jaw is aching.

"When you notice that your hand has become numb, your hand lifts up and touches your jaw. When your numb hand touches your jaw, the numbness is transferred to the jaw and soaks into the mouth, bringing relief. The numb comfort soaks into the jaw and your jaw becomes quite comfortable."

Using Subconscious Associations for Better Results

The painkillers novocaine and lidocaine usually take about five minutes to create numbness. Over the years I have noticed that from the initial suggestion of hypnotic anesthesia to the experience of numbness, my clients usually needed about the same amount of time. If a client has had chemo-anesthesia in the past, they are conditioned to it taking a few minutes before numbness is experienced. In hypnosis, that association can actually make the numbing process take longer than it needs to. To test this premise, I have suggested to clients that the hypnotic anesthesia works faster than typical chemo-anesthesia and, sure enough, they were then able to achieve numbness in a shorter period of time.

Discovering that the time to establish the glove anesthesia was approximately the same as the time for an injection of novocaine to take effect got me thinking about other associations that might be helpful in creating hypnotic analgesia and anesthesia. My experience has shown that people respond better to these techniques when they have an attitude of having already succeeded and feeling grateful for their success. Knowing this, I have developed a practice of first facilitating my clients into strong, associated feelings of success and gratitude before using techniques like glove anesthesia.

To help the client create a feeling of success, I ask them to remember something they have done successfully in the past and then step into that experience and get in touch with all those good feelings. For the feeling of gratitude, I ask them to think about someone in their life that they really appreciate. This could be a friend, a loved one, or even a favorite pet. I then invite them to get in touch with the feeling of being grateful for having them in their life. The feeling of success sets them up to create an outcome that they can feel grateful for, and the feeling of gratitude puts them in the state of having already achieved that outcome. That is the optimal attitude for glove anesthesia, or any other pain control technique for that matter.

Patrick Singleton, developer of the Creative NLP™ (Neuro-Linguistic Programming) Training and instructor at the Hypnotherapy Academy, suggests we teach the client how to "anchor" these resources. Anchoring means establishing a signal or trigger that activates a feeling state rapidly. In the next glove anesthesia process, you will see how to help your clients get in touch with and anchor these resources for better results.

Glove Anesthesia with an Icy Numbing Solution
This version of the glove anesthesia technique uses the client's subconscious associations to cold by having them imagine dipping their hand into a bucket full of an icy numbing solution. Many people have experienced their hands going partially or completely numb from the cold. By including suggestions for cold and remembering experiences of cold things like playing in the snow, you will help the client to recreate the numb feeling. Because cold is an uncomfortable sensation for most people though, do not spend too much time on it. Suggest that the cold sensation is brief and turns into comfortable numbness quickly.

In the following process we show the client how to combine the success and gratitude resources with their associations to cold to effectively erase their perception of pain. After inducing hypnosis, deepening, and testing, continue as follows.

> "(Person's name), take a moment now and think about something you have done or been part of in the past that was a success. It doesn't matter if it was a day ago, a month ago, or years ago. What matters is that it was a success and you feel proud to have accomplished it. When you have found something that you did that you succeeded at, nod your head."

Wait for client to nod, then continue.

> "Good. Now just step into that experience fully and completely and get in touch with all the good feelings of that success moment. When you've really got those good feelings of success and being proud of yourself, smile so I know you are feeling good."

Wait for client to smile, then continue. Now that the client is experiencing the feeling of success, you will show them how to anchor that feeling so they can easily get back to it in the future.

> "Now open your mouth and take a deep breath to feel even more of those good feelings. As you breathe, and the feeling grows stronger, press your left hand's index finger and thumb together firmly. Pressing your index finger and thumb together like this is a signal to feel powerful success feelings immediately."

Wait for client to breathe and anchor the success resource, then continue. When the client breathes in another breath, you can also add, "That's right, breathe it in and the feeling gets stronger."

> "That's right. Now let go of that time, and as you release the finger and thumb you can hold on to those success feelings."

Wait for client to separate their finger and thumb, then continue.

> "Now think about someone in your life that you really appreciate. It could be a friend, a loved one, or a favorite pet. When you have done that, nod your head."

Wait for client to nod, then continue.

> "Alright, get in touch with the gratitude you have for them and their being in your life. Let the feeling of appreciation fill you. And when you're really filled with the feelings of appreciation and gratitude, smile so that I know you've got it."

Wait for client to smile, then continue. Now add the feelings of gratitude to the anchor for success, so that they can use the same anchor to get both feelings at once.

> "That's right. Now take another good, deep breath, and as those good feelings grow stronger now, press your left hand's index finger and thumb together just like before and really feel the gratitude you have for them. As you do, also notice those strong feelings of success coming right back to you. Pressing your index finger and thumb together like this is a signal to feel gratitude and appreciation and success strongly and immediately. You can use this signal any time you would like. Just press your index finger and thumb together just as you're doing right now and

those good feelings come right back to you. Now keep those good feelings as you release the finger and thumb."

Wait for client to separate their finger and thumb, then continue. Now begin with the icy numbing solution.

"Now imagine that there is a bucket sitting over here on the right side of the chair. Imagine it contains a bluish icy numbing solution. In a moment you're going to pick up your right hand and dip the hand all the way into that icy numbing solution. When you dip your hand into that icy numbing solution, your hand first grows cold and tingly. Then, your hand will soak up a layer of this numbing solution, and quickly grow comfortably numb. Your hand will continue to soak up that numbing solution and lose sensation until your hand is completely numb. To make this really easy, please put pleasant liquid saliva in your mouth now. Nod your head when you've done that."

Wait for client to nod, then continue.

"Now repeat the following out loud: 'I am the master of my mind. My body responds to my thoughts.'"

Wait for client to repeat the suggestion.

"Now take a deep breath and press your left hand's index finger and thumb together and you feel those strong feelings of success and gratitude coming right back to you. That's right. Now smile and repeat: 'As I put my hand in the numbing solution, my hand quickly becomes anesthetized.'"

Wait for client to repeat the suggestion.

> "Good. Now lift your right hand up, (person's name), even though it feels very heavy. Lift it over the side of the chair and dip it into that numbing solution."

The client lifts their right hand up and hangs it over the arm of the chair. When they do this, the shift in blood flow causes a tingling sensation in the hand. Knowing this, we suggest that the numbness begins with a tingling sensation. When the client begins to feel the tingling in their hand, they will assume it's because they are responding to your suggestion, and that will build confidence, which will help them become more responsive to subsequent suggestions for more complete numbness.

In this next part of the script we mention that the numbness is like having novocaine—another association to numbness. Before using this technique, find out if the client has an allergy to novocaine, and if so, omit this reference to avoid any conscious mind objection that might lessen their response.

> "That's right. First the solution feels kind of cold, then tingly, and numbing. Notice the tingling sensation beginning in your right hand now as it is beginning to grow numb. Soon your right hand is numb, wooden, almost stiff, and all sensation is vanishing. Your hand is like a sponge. It soaks up fluid through your skin, your pores. Soaking up this magical, healing, numbing solution.
>
> Now put more liquid saliva in your mouth and say out loud, 'My right hand is now anesthetized.'"

Wait for client to repeat the suggestion.

> "Now slowly swirl your hand around in the numbing solution. Your hand is becoming more and more numb now as it's soaking up more of the numbing solution. When your hand is filled with that numb feeling, it begins to slowly float up. The hand is filling, soaking up that numbing solution, and after it gets that numb, stiff, wooden-like feeling, that right hand will start to float up. It's just as if novocaine is soaking in through the pores of the skin on your right hand and you're losing all sensation in your hand now. As soon as the hand becomes numb, it starts to float up. And as it floats up, it becomes more and more numb."

Continue with suggestions of numbness and loss of sensation while you wait for the client's arm to begin lifting up. Be encouraging of any movement. When their hand has clearly begun to float up as suggested, that's your sign that they have achieved numbness in the hand. Now, to help the client build confidence in their ability to transfer that numbness to other parts of their body, have them transfer it first to one side of their face, and then to the other side, and then back to the hand. Continue as follows:

> "And now you are going to transfer all this numbness by letting the hand float up until it touches your right cheek and jaw. When your hand touches your jaw, the numbness in your hand transfers into the right side of your face, just as if you had novocaine."

Wait until the client's hand touches their face, then continue.

> "Good. You can press the hand into the face now. You're just transferring and filling the face and jaw with the numbness. The whole right side of your face starts to feel numb and comfortable, more and more, with each passing moment. Even the skin of the face starts to feel tingly and become numb. When the numbness is transferred to the right side of your face, your arm will fall limply to your side."

Wait until the client drops their arm to their side, then continue.

> "That's good. And notice the comfort increasing with each easy breath that you take, each easy heartbeat. Every time your heart beats there's more of that numbing solution moving into your face. It moves into the jaw and the teeth. You can even try to move your face a little bit and notice how different it feels, puffy and numb. As you start to notice it, nod your head."

Client nods their head.

> "Very good. In a moment, I'm going to snap my fingers three times. When I snap my fingers three times, all that numbness is going to transfer to the left side of the face. It'll go into the left side of the face, the jaw, into the teeth and the left side of the tongue."

Snap your fingers three times.

> "Good. All that pleasant numbness is transferring now to the left side of the face. The left side of your face, jaw, teeth, and tongue are losing all sensation and growing numb now."

Wait a minute to give the client time to transfer the numbness.

> "Very good. And now I'm going to snap my fingers three times again and all the numbness will go back into your right hand. As I snap my fingers, your mouth, teeth, and jaw regain their normal sensation."

Snap your fingers three times.

> "That's it. All the numbing solution goes back to your right hand. Your mouth regains normal sensation as the numbness moves back to your hand now. When the numbness is back in your hand, nod your head."

Client nods head.

> "Now that the numbness is in your hand, move your hand up and over to the bucket."

Wait for client to move their hand over the imaginary bucket, then continue.

> "Take a good breath and let all the solution leave your hand, draining the solution back into the bucket. All that numbing solution is going to go back into the bucket. Let it all drain out. And as it all drains out, normal sensation comes back to your hand. Normal sensation comes back. When all of the numbing solution has drained back into the bucket, your hand will come back to rest at your side. Imagine putting a lid on the bucket and putting it in a special place for you to use any time you like."

Now program the client for increasing responsiveness each time they practice hypnosis and glove anesthesia.

> "(Person's name), what you are about to hear is the truth about you. Each time you go into hypnosis, you go faster and deeper than the time before. You respond even more profoundly, than you did the time before. Every time you practice your hypnotic techniques you find yourself reaching even greater levels of success and satisfaction. Your creative subconscious intelligence knows exactly how to help you feel comfortable and heal, and so it does this for you now, and every time you practice hypnosis. Every day and in every way, you are getting better and better now. (Person's name), feelings of strength and confidence grow as you practice hypnosis daily. You are making positive use of your inner resources and that pleases you. This is not because I say so, but because it is your natural ability to do so."

De-hypnotize. Remember to energize your voice a bit and enliven the tempo as you bring them out of hypnosis.

> "In a moment I'll count from one up to five and you'll bring yourself up and out of hypnosis.
>
> One… Peacefully, calmly, easily, and gently bringing yourself up and out of hypnosis.
>
> Two… Each muscle and nerve in your body feels loose, limp and relaxed. You feel good!
>
> Three… You look forward to returning to hypnosis. It feels good to know you have successfully used your mind power to control your bodily sensations.

Number Four… You're feeling wonderfully good about your new powers, your power of mind and the ability to control your body's sensations. On the next number your eyes will open and you'll be fully aware in every way.

Five… Eyes open, fully aware. Stretch and smile."

CHAPTER 12

Amelioration by Dissociation

Chronic pain is often treated with analgesics and psychotropics. While many people experience temporary relief from their pain with this treatment, the side effects are well documented. Analgesics can be addictive, and psychotropics can cause mood changes and a lack of mental clarity. Hypnotic pain control methods can be just as effective while having no negative side effects whatsoever. In this chapter I will show you how to use dissociation to reduce and even eliminate pain.

Pain Relief by Dissociation
Dissociation means getting distance or disconnecting from something. For pain relief purposes, we help the client to create a *perceptual distance from their pain by dissociating from their own body.* You do this by having the client imagine themselves floating out of their body and going to a pleasant place of comfort and healing. I have found the dissociation method very useful for any type or intensity of pain.

Before inducing hypnosis, ask the client to tell you about a pleasant place, real or imaginary, where they feel comfortable and at ease. Get some details so that you can guide them to their pleasant place and make it vivid for them. The place they choose should be a place appropriate for healing and pain control work. A beach is a common choice, so we will use that in our example. As usual, you should check for the appropriateness of the imagery you intend to use. After choosing a pleasant place, inducing hypnosis, deepening, and testing, proceed as follows:

> "(Person's name), I'm now going to show you how to feel more comfortable. You told me earlier about a place you would rather be, instead of here in the hospital. I want you to start thinking about that place now."

If the place was not determined prior to hypnosis, you can easily prompt the client in this way.

> "I'm sure there's somewhere else you'd rather be than here in the hospital. Think about a place that is calming to you. Maybe a beach, or a mountain meadow, or a place you like to go when you're on vacation. This can be a real or an imaginary place. When you think of a place you would rather be, say a few words to describe it for me."

You don't want them to say too much here. Having to verbalize more than a few words tends to bring them into their left-brain and out of the experience a little. So here we continue with the beach example.

> "Okay, now to help you get there, and to help yourself feel better, imagine, sense, and feel that you are safely lifting up and floating to that place. Thinking

> of lifting up and floating away causes your body to become pleasantly numb. Easily and gently lifting up and drifting and floating safely away from the hospital and toward your peaceful, pleasant place where you feel comfortable and at ease."

Remember the last time you had an endorphin high? What did it feel like? Most people report a kind of ecstatic floating feeling accompanying an endorphin release. When vividly imagining floating or flying while in hypnosis, many people experience a release of endorphins. This helps create the physical feeling of floating, which will make the experience more real for them. More importantly, it also helps reduce their sensitivity to pain. Continue as follows:

> "(Person's name), imagine lifting up and away from the hospital, floating toward that pleasant place and feeling free. Feeling free and easy as you float closer and closer to that peaceful, pleasant place where you feel so comfortable. Just keep floating closer now, and when you're there, just nod your head."

Wait for client to nod, then continue.

> "Very good. Floating all the way to that beach that you told me about. Now put yourself at the beach. Sense the warm sand on the bottom of your feet. Think about and imagine the smell of the fresh sea air and the open sky above you. Fill in the details and make it vivid and real for yourself. Find the right place to rest and relax here on the beach, and when you have done that, just nod your head."

Wait for client to nod, then continue.

"That's right. By resting here on the beach you feel more and more comfortable now. The rest and relaxation you feel on the beach helps you feel good and comfortable in every way. You stay here on the beach and feel better and better with every easy breath you breathe. With each passing moment you discover greater peace and comfort here on the beach. Everything you hear takes you deeper into the experience of being at the beach.

You may even notice that you hear the water lapping at the shore as the gentle waves come in and out. You may even notice the foam from the waves floating in and out on the water. Every new detail you notice takes you deeper and deeper relaxed and you feel more and more comfortable with each passing moment. So breathe easily and just be here now while I'm quiet."

You have a few options now. If you're working with a client who is currently undergoing a medical procedure, you can have the client stay in their pleasant place until the procedure is complete and suggest that they feel comfortable during and after the work. If the pain is from an injury that is healing, you can suggest that they stay in their pleasant place for ten to twenty minutes while the body repairs itself. In both cases, suggest that when they come out of hypnosis, they come back into their body, bringing the good feelings of peace and comfort with them.

Watching the Body Give Up the Pain
This technique combines the dissociation method with the dilution method discussed earlier. Start by having the client imagine themselves outside of their body. Then have them

watch the pain drain out of their body, from a comfortable distance, using the dilution technique. After the pain has drained out of the body and comfort is regained, the client then returns to their body. In the following example, the client is still in the hospital and is recovering from shoulder surgery they had earlier that morning. After inducing hypnosis, deepening, and testing, continue as follows:

> "Alright (person's name), for just a few moments I want you to analyze the pain in your shoulder. Tune in to the pain and notice what color it is. When you have the color, say it out loud."

Some clients will experience slightly more pain when they tune in to the feeling to get the color. That is okay because it will only be for a few moments. Wait until the client says the color, then continue. In this example, the client says, "Red."

> "Red. Very good. Now (person's name), I want you to see yourself from a very different perspective. Imagine floating up and out of your body. Float over toward the doorway of this room. When you're standing in the doorway turn and look back at yourself lying there on the bed. Imagine this as vividly as you can.
>
> Look around you. Look and notice the things around you. Look above and below, side to side, and as you do, realize that by being outside of your body, you are also outside and away from the pain you were having before.
>
> Now look back again and see your body lying in the bed. Lying there with the pain in the shoulder. When you have done that, nod your head."

Wait for client to nod, then continue.

> "That's right. You're doing really well. Now, you've got to get that pain out of that shoulder. As you look at your body lying there, see the red pain in the shoulder. Now imagine that the red pain is beginning to drain down, out of the shoulder, down the arm. See the red pain just draining and moving down, down the arm, down now toward the elbow."

With the dilution technique, you want to let the pain representation drain away from the center of the body and the painful area and out the end of the nearest extremity. In the case of shoulder surgery, their arm is likely to be immobilized and bandaged to their chest. So instead of going all the way to the hand, which would bring the pain back toward the center of the body, we have them drain the pain out of the elbow.

> "As the red color is moving away from the shoulder and down the arm, the pain is moving down the arm with it. Because the red color is moving down the arm, the pain is moving down to the elbow. Watch as the red painful feeling moves all the way down to the elbow now. As you see that happening, all the pain is moving completely into the elbow.
>
> Now imagine and see the red pain beginning to drain out the tip of the elbow. Just watch as all the red pain drains out now. Just letting it all drain out.
>
> That's right. And because all the red is draining out completely, your shoulder and arm begin to feel much more comfortable now. You see yourself feeling

> much better. When all the red is completely gone, and you're feeling comfortable, just nod your head."

Wait for client to nod, then continue.

> "Good. Now just watch all the red color drain off onto the floor and evaporate. As it evaporates, you notice that you're already feeling much more comfortable.
>
> Now I want you to find a part of the body that is comfortable and give that comfortable feeling a color. When you've done that, say the color out loud and tell me which part of the body it's in."

Wait for client to answer, then continue. For this example, let's say the client answers that the comfortable feeling is green and that it's in their legs.

> "Green. Excellent. Now watch as the green comfort expands from the legs up through the hips and torso and into the back. The green color moving up through the body into the back brings that comfortable, good feeling up along with it. See the pleasant green color moving up the back and into the shoulder now. Because the green comfortable feeling is moving up to the shoulder, your shoulder feels more and more comfortable now. When the shoulder is filled with the green color and you're feeling good, nod your head.

Wait for client to nod, then continue.

> "In that case, you can begin moving back toward your body now. As you get closer, see the shoulder filled with green comfort. That green, comfortable feeling is

in, and all around, your shoulder. To feel even more comfort, get back into your body and notice the peaceful, pleasant green in your shoulder. When you are back in your body and feeling that comfortable feeling in your shoulder, nod your head."

Wait for client to nod, then continue. Now you can continue with therapeutic suggestions and healing imagery. When you count the client out of hypnosis, be sure to include suggestions for accelerated healing and continuing comfort in the areas where they had pain.

CHAPTER 13

Supporting the Immune System and Self-Hypnosis Training Methods

Supporting the immune system is a lifestyle choice. It is choosing to eat the right organic foods, lean meats, and a lot more fruits and vegetables. It is cutting down on the consumption of sugar and alcohol. It is choosing to exercise and get outside in the sunshine. It is choosing to reduce contact with man-made chemicals like those found in some paints, perfumes, carpet, household cleaning products, and so on. And it is choosing not to expose the body to toxic thoughts.

Toxic thoughts have only two sources. They can either originate within ourselves or come from other people. Pessimistic and gloomy thoughts, angry and violent thoughts, regretful and fearful thoughts are all toxic and suppress the body's natural healing ability. It is, therefore, important for the sick and injured to understand that they have the right to remove themselves from negative environments and the God-given ability to improve the quality of their own thinking habits.

Every time you hypnotize a client and program positive therapeutic suggestions, the foundation of optimism is strengthened for them. Additionally, you are teaching them the vocabulary of positive change. Every time you hypnotize a client, and every time they practice self-hypnosis, their immune system (which receives its marching orders from the autonomic nervous system) receives instructions to boost its function. By teaching a client how to enter into the profound relaxation of deep trance a few times each day, their body gets into the habit of switching out of stress and survival mode (sympathetic nervous system) and into health-restoring mode (parasympathetic nervous system).

The Ethics of Self-Hypnosis
Supporting the immune system through the daily practice of self-hypnosis and intentional autosuggestion is an integral part of the medical hypnotherapy strategy. The mental Law of Repetitive Effect tells us that the more you are exposed to an idea, the more likely it is that you will accept and act upon it. Combining this repetition with the bypassing of the critical faculty through self-hypnosis makes a very powerful self-healing method.

We have a saying in this work that you should *never work harder than your client.* This statement has a double meaning. First, it reminds us to teach the client to do their own healing work. And second, it serves as a reminder to be ethical in the use of power.

For the good of ourselves and our clients, it is important to understand that it is always the client who heals themselves. As hypnotherapists, we coach, guide, and teach the client how to best make use of their own inner resources to regain balance and heal themselves. A healthy therapeutic relationship includes creating a psychic collaboration where our mind power is united with the client's, as teammates, for the sole purpose of their healing or pain control. To approach the client with the idea that you are here to heal them is unethical because it introduces an unhealthy imbalance into the relationship, as if you are superior to them. Perhaps the best way to maintain the proper balance of power is to require your clients to practice self-hypnosis between visits with you. And remember: never work harder than your client.

Saturate the Mind with Intentional Autosuggestion
Methods to saturate the mind with high-quality thoughts have been used for thousands of years to bring about positive change in behavior and to produce greater well-being. In the East, you might see a Buddhist or Hindu meditator sitting in the lotus position with one hand resting in their lap and the other holding a mala. The mala is long strand of 108 beads with a large knot at the end. The meditator, sitting peacefully, usually with eyes closed, whispers an invocation over and over and over while dragging the beads over one of their fingers to keep track of the count. In the West you can see a Catholic using a rosary during prayers as a counting device as well. In both examples, the use of a counting device enables the user to stay focused on the invocation and not be distracted by counting the number of times they've said each prayer. Counting engages the conscious mind, which weakens the trance state. By letting the beads do the counting, the conscious mind can remain relaxed and the client's subconscious stays more open and receptive to positive ideas.

Emile Coué said that *every thought entirely filling our mind becomes true for us and tends to transform itself into action.* He advised his clients to tie knots in a piece of medium weight string for use as a counting device. He would then have them induce self-hypnosis twice a day and repeat a general affirmation such as, "Every day, in every way, I am getting better and better" at least twenty times, using the knotted string to keep count.

This kind of generalized incremental affirmation is now known as a generalized Couism. Coué argued that we could try to address every single problem or symptom individually until the cows come home and we may still never actually address the real heart of the issue. By making the affirmation general with a phrase like, "in every way," you can just let the client's inner creative mind do its perfect work and go about improving whatever needs improving. And by making the affirmation incremental, it becomes more believable and therefore acceptable to the critical faculty.

Today at the Academy we teach hypnotherapists learning medical hypnosis to coach their clients in the following self-hypnosis strategy.

Have clients practice self-hypnosis twice daily. The effects of hypnosis are accumulative and progressive, so the more often they practice, the better their subconscious will respond.

Teach clients to use a counting device. Either a string with knots, or a wrist-length mala, which commonly has eighteen beads, will suffice. It is easiest to teach a new client how to use the counting device before inducing trance.

Caution clients that they are never to use a hypnosis audio while operating machinery or driving an automobile. If a client wants to focus on their therapeutic suggestions while driving, you can create a recording of all the programming without the induction and deepening. When making such an audio recording, use a high-energy voice and change around the order of the suggestions and add suggestions that they are alert and focused while they

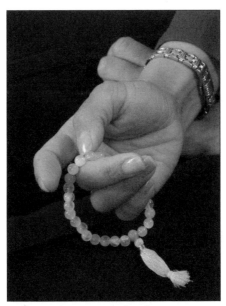

Affirmation counting beads

listen. Coach the client to repeat each suggestion out loud after you. Every so often, people who trained with me and who have a musical background creatively convert the positive programming into a kind of sing-a-long for the client to use as a non-trance programming audio.

Instruct clients to avoid the use of stimulants like tea or coffee before self-hypnosis.

The length of the audio should be about fifteen minutes or less. I have made hundreds and hundreds of personalized audios for clients and they have had major breakthroughs, healed faster, and felt better. The only critical feedback I have gotten was that the audio was too long. So I streamlined the content and they got the same results in less time. If the audio is twenty to thirty minutes long and you ask them to listen to it two or three times a day, that's too much of a time commitment for most people. The methods in this book are designed with time consideration in mind.

Instruct clients to sit or lie down somewhere comfortable where they will not be disturbed by people or telephones, and loosen any tight or restricting clothing. If sitting, they should keep their back straight and head slightly tilted down about a half inch. This tends to take some of the strain out of the neck muscles. If lying down, have them lie flat with their arms at their sides and legs uncrossed. If they tend to fall asleep lying down, have them sit up for hypnosis.

Condition clients to be able to induce self-hypnosis using a simple signal. The most effective time to anchor a signal is at the peak of the state you wish to anchor. A client will typically be deepest in the trance state toward the end of the session, so that is the best time to teach them how to induce self-hypnosis.

Example Script for Teaching Self-Hypnosis
After inducing and deepening trance, teach the client how to induce self-hypnosis and saturate their mind with autosuggestion as follows.

> "In a moment I will show you an effective method for practicing self-hypnosis. Because this method is so powerful, when you practice it on your own, you will go just as deep into hypnosis as you are right now, and your subconscious will be just as responsive to your positive programming.
>
> Every morning, and every evening, you help yourself heal by directing your powerful inner resources using this method. In a moment you will open your eyes and find a nice spot, high above you, to stare at. You will then take three deep breaths. As you exhale the third deep breath, whisper the words 'sleep now' and just close your eyes. The words 'sleep now' are

your signal to enter the deep, pleasant, healing state of hypnosis. When you give yourself the signal 'sleep now' your eyelids instantly close down and you are then in a pleasant state of hypnosis. You then easily and effectively direct your inner creative intelligence to accelerate your healing.

Alright, (person's name), open your eyes now and find a nice spot high above you to stare at. Take your first deep breath and exhale slowly."

Pause while client takes a deep breath.

"Good, keep staring at that nice spot and take your second deep breath and exhale slowly."

Pause while client takes a deep breath.

"Good, now take your third deep breath, and as you exhale slowly, give yourself the 'sleep now' signal by saying it out loud. Then just close your eyes."

Pause while client takes the last deep breath. After they close their eyes, continue.

"That's right. Notice how you are already going deep into hypnosis. Now the next step is to relax your eyelids so much that they just won't work. By relaxing your eyelids so much that they won't work, you put yourself into the perfect depth of hypnosis so your autosuggestions successfully plant themselves in the fertile soil of your creative subconscious mind. When you have relaxed your eyelids so much that they just won't work, test them and find that you have been successful."

Wait for client to test their eyelids, then continue.

> "That's right. You have achieved the right type of hypnotic state, and because you have, all the systems of your body reset themselves to function optimally. All the systems of your body now work in perfect harmony. (Person's name), your powerful immune system keeps you safe and healthy now.
>
> (Person's name), it's time to give your subconscious creative intelligence directions to accelerate your healing. What you are about to say to yourself makes a vivid and permanent impression on your subconscious mind. Because of this, your subconscious mind immediately acts on all of these beneficial ideas. Using your counting beads, repeat the following statement out loud with each bead until you finish the round. Speak in a soft but confident tone and say, 'Every day, in every way, I am getting better and better now.'"

It will take a few minutes for your client to complete the round of beads. You can make use of that time by putting yourself in a light trance and repeating the suggestion with them in your mind a few times, replacing the word 'I' with their name: "Every day, in every way, (person's name) is getting better and better." Then, while the client is still repeating the therapeutic suggestion, vividly picture them in your mind as completely healed of their health issue. Fill yourself with feelings of joy and gratitude for their complete healing.

After the client has finished the round of eighteen beads, instruct them to do another round using a specialized therapeutic suggestion. Say, for example, that your client is healing congestive heart failure. This is a condition where

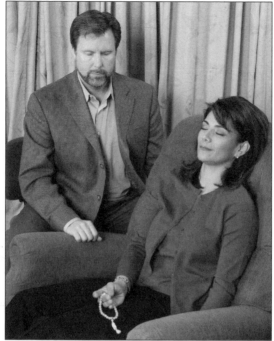

Generating a noetigenic field of healing probability while client uses counting beads

the heart muscle has stretched and a full contraction of the atrium and ventricle is not occurring. In this case, you could instruct the client as follows:

> **"Good work. Now I want you to go through another round of beads, and this time, I want you to say, 'Every day, in every way, my healing heart beats more strongly and efficiently now.'"**

As before, you can help by repeating the affirmation with them in your mind and then holding the image of them healed vividly in your mind while you wait for them to finish. After the client has finished the round, continue as follows:

> "Now (person's name), vividly imagine a day in your life after your healing is complete. It's the near future and you are doing something that you enjoy because you are healthy now. Make it vivid and real and get the good feelings that you would have if you were really there right now. Then after you have created this mental movie and have all the good feelings, including gratitude for your healing, nod your head."

Wait for client to nod their head. This should take them a minute or two. If they nod their head after just a few seconds, they didn't take enough time to really see the details and bathe in the good feelings, so have them review the imagery again in greater detail. After the client nods their head, continue as follows:

> "Now it's time to take yourself out of hypnosis. Count from one up to five and slowly bring yourself completely out of hypnosis. When you reach the number five, open your eyes. You are then alert and fully aware, feeling good in every way. Now (person's name), begin counting and bring yourself out of hypnosis feeling rested and refreshed."

Supporting the Immune System with Active Relaxation Training

The active relaxation process is just like a progressive relaxation, except that as we go through the regions of the body we ask the client first to contract the muscles strongly before relaxing them. While this may seem counterintuitive, it actually helps create a deeper level of relaxation than would be achieved by just passively relaxing the muscles. This works because of the muscle reflex known as autogenic inhibition, which causes the muscle to relax immediately following a contraction. This relaxation reflex helps release habitual tension that may not be released in a progressive relaxation based on guided imagery alone. The profound relaxation achievable by this method accelerates healing and recovery and helps the body to bring itself back into balance.

Explain the process to your client before beginning. Then, after inducing hypnosis, proceed as follows:

> "Now let's begin the active relaxation process we talked about. In a moment we will begin moving through each part of your body. For each part, I will have you tense up the muscles and hold the tension for a few seconds. Then you'll take a breath in and then say 'relax' out loud and exhale as you let go of all the tension. As you do this, I want you to tune in to the muscles closely and notice what the tension feels like and then notice how good the relaxation feels when you release.
>
> Alright, now tense up your left foot, calf, and thigh. Tense them hard and notice what the tension feels like. In a moment I want you to take a breath in and then say the word 'relax' and exhale as you slowly release all the tension from your left foot, calf, and thigh muscles. Saying 'relax' is your signal to release all tension. Okay, (person's name), take a breath in, then say 'relax' out loud and exhale."

Wait for client to exhale, then continue.

> "That's right. Very slowly let all the tension out of your left foot, calf, and thigh. As you release the muscles, allow a warm, relaxing sensation to come into your left leg. Notice how the relaxation feels."

Pause about ten seconds while the client relaxes.

> "Now (person's name), tense up your right foot, calf, and thigh muscles. Tense them hard and notice what the tension feels like. Hold that tension for a few moments and then take a breath in, and then say 'relax' and exhale."

Wait for client to exhale, then continue.

> "That's right. Just slowly letting all the tension out of your right foot, calf, and thigh now. As you release the muscles, allow a warm, relaxing sensation to come into your right leg. Notice how the relaxation feels."

Pause about ten seconds while the client relaxes.

> "Very good. Now, make a tight fist with your left hand and then tense up your entire left arm. Notice what the tension feels like."

Pause a few seconds, then continue.

> "Okay, take a breath in, then say 'relax' in your mind and exhale. As you exhale, slowly let all the tension out of your left hand and arm. As you release the muscles, allow a warm, relaxing feeling to come into your left arm and hand now and notice how good that feels.

Pause about ten seconds while the client relaxes.

> "Good. And now make a fist with your right hand and then tense up your entire right arm. Notice what the tension feels like."

Pause a few seconds, then continue.

> "Okay, take a breath in, then say 'relax' in your mind and exhale. As you exhale, slowly let all the tension out of your right hand and arm. As you release the muscles, allow a warm, relaxing feeling to come into your right arm and hand now and notice how good that feels."

Pause about ten seconds while the client relaxes.

> "Very good. Now take another breath in, and hold it as you tense up your belly muscles. Notice what the tension feels like."

Pause a few seconds, then continue.

> "Okay, now say 'relax' in your mind and exhale. As you exhale, slowly let all the tension out of your belly muscles. As you release the muscles, allow that warm, relaxing sensation of peace and calm to spread into your belly and notice how good that feels."

Pause about ten seconds while the client relaxes.

> "Very good. Now tense up your shoulder and neck muscles. Lift up your shoulders and tense them hard. Notice what the tension feels like."

Pause a few seconds, then continue.

> "Alright, now take in a breath, then say 'relax' and exhale. As you exhale, let your shoulders fall and let all the tension out of your shoulders and neck.

> As you release the muscles, allow a warm, pleasant sensation to come into your neck and shoulders and notice how good that feels."

Pause about ten seconds while the client relaxes.

> "You are going deeper and deeper into hypnotic relaxation. Because you are releasing all the old tension from your body, all the systems of your body work in perfect harmony more and more now.
>
> Now tense up your facial muscles. Scrunch up your face and notice what the tension feels like."

Pause a few seconds, then continue.

> "That's right, now to go even deeper into hypnotic relaxation, take another breath, then say 'relax' and exhale. As you exhale, totally let go of all tension in your face. Relax your jaw muscles, allowing a slight space between your teeth. Expand the warm, pleasant feeling into all the muscles of your face and jaw and notice how good that feels."

Pause about ten seconds while the client relaxes.

> "That's right. Enjoy the complete peace and relaxation you have created now. You are at peace with yourself. Your body responds to your positive and healing thoughts. Whenever you want to relax, you know what to do. You tense up the muscles for just a moment, take a breath, then say 'relax' and exhale as you release the tension, and allow your muscles to turn loose. That's right. It's very easy for you to relax completely now."

Vagus Nerve Stimulation with Diaphragmatic Breathing
The tenth cranial nerve, called the vagus nerve, helps regulate autonomic nervous system functions. Vagus means "wanderer" and this nerve does wander throughout the body. It originates in the base of the lower brain and travels down the neck into the torso, connecting with major organs like the heart and lungs along the way. It continues down through the diaphragm and abdominal area and terminates at the rectum. Deep diaphragmatic breathing activates the parasympathetic nervous system by stimulating the vagus nerve. This boosts immune function, regulates digestion and heart rate, relaxes the body, and promotes many other beneficial body processes.

A full diaphragmatic breath begins by intentionally directing your inhale into the belly area first in order to engage the diaphragm. The inhale is as long and full as it can be while still being comfortable. When exhaling, the chest falls first and the belly last. Inhale through the nose in order to warm and filter incoming air, and exhale slowly through the mouth. Slightly pursing the lips helps to control the slow exhale. Exhaling out the mouth also helps to discharge the old air more completely.

Diaphragmatic breathing can be used as a deepening or as a non-trance technique for relaxation and stress relief. Coach the client through a cycle of nine breaths. As you coach them in the correct technique, give them therapeutic suggestions that promote feelings of safety, peace, and healthy well-being. After completing the cycle of nine diaphragmatic breaths, tell them to just breathe normally, then continue the session with other therapeutic suggestions and healing imagery appropriate to their hypnotherapy goals.

CHAPTER 14

An Introduction to Noetigenesis™ and Developing Your Healing Presence

Throughout this book I have presented many effective techniques and example scripts; however, it is not the techniques themselves, nor just the words spoken, that make healing and transformation manifest. There is no magic in the words, and the techniques are simply examples of utilizing the deeper resources of the human mind. The words and techniques are merely the vehicle that provides a link between a healing presence and a healing potential.

Over the last three decades I have been blessed to witness many human miracles. People written off as permanently disabled have gotten out of my hypnosis chair to walk again with ease. Those said to have only weeks to live because of cancer integrate hypnotherapy into their healing strategy and go on to live for years. Yet hypnosis is not a panacea. Some people just don't respond as well as others. But what makes the difference? Why do some people experience miraculous transformation in their health and in their lives while others experience only mediocre results?

Part of what makes a person ready for a healing experience was covered in Chapter Eight, with overcoming the roadblocks to healing and pain relief. But real transformation requires more than just the absence of blocks. The mystery of human miracles requires more inquiry. After years of late nights researching ancient wisdom traditions and modern scientific works, I came to see a common thread running through both. This commonality helped me to understand the miraculous transformations I have witnessed.

Healing happens most rapidly when two or more minds join to create a perfect thought-union with the singular purpose of seeing the client as joyfully whole. More than the skillful use of words and techniques to remove the blocks to wellness, this synergistic joining of minds is the aim of the hypnotherapeutic encounter.

Admittedly, this understanding of healing, hypnotherapy and human miracles is a bit esoteric. Something "esoteric" is typically understood by an initiated few, or is beyond the average understanding. Rightfully so, the understanding that healing happens when we create a thought-union of joyful wholeness is not the average definition. Consensual reality, the common agreement about what is real, says that if you can stick a fork in it, it exists, and if you cannot, it does not. Human miracles cannot be explained when peering through the lens of consensual reality. When we look beyond consensual reality we discover that our minds are all linked together by a unifying field of intelligence. This thought-connecting field joins everyone at the subconscious and superconscious levels, which means that a thought from one person has the remarkable ability to transfer itself to another person in an instant. It also means that any thought I hold in my mind is also available to your mind.

The Science of Consciousness

Researchers who study consciousness scientifically are now explaining how hypnotherapy influences human miracles. An excellent example is an experiment done by William Braud and Marilyn Schlitz in which they wanted to determine if imagery held in the mind of one person could influence the physiology of another person at a distance.

The experiment was conducted with one person, the subject, sitting alone in a room. The subject's vital signs, including skin moisture, were closely monitored for the duration of the test period. While they sat, they were exposed to various neutral visual and auditory stimuli.

At the same time, another person, the influencer, sat in a separate room. Precautions were taken to make sure that no form of physical communication was possible between the two people. At various times during the test period, the influencer was instructed to use mental imagery to attempt to influence the subject's physiology, sometimes to calm them and sometimes to stimulate them. The subject, of course, had no idea when this would happen.

Of the 337 people participating in the experiment, 271 were subjects, 62 were influencers, and four were experimenters. Before the experiment, it was believed that the influencer would be able to affect the physiology of the subject five percent of the time. Instead, the influencers achieved an amazing forty percent success rate at influencing the subject's biological functions at a distance!

This means that we communicate in some way other than the five senses (no fork needed). Cleve Backster, researcher, author of numerous books on the subject of nonverbal communication, and longtime student of hypnotism, calls this kind of non-physical communication "primary perception." Backster first scientifically established primary perception in 1966 by hooking up a plant to a polygraph machine. He found that specific emotional imagery generated by a human caused a measurable response in the plant being monitored by the polygraph.

Later in an experiment conducted in June of 1980, Backster tested human leukocytes for primary perception and found that the emotions of the donor could cause a measurable response in their leukocytes at a distance. He put the donor's white blood cells in a tube and inserted electrodes to monitor them. The monitored leukocytes showed a measurable reaction when the donor, at a distance of fifteen feet, experienced a strong emotion.

Backster's book, *Primary Perception,* which I recommend to anyone in the healing arts, tells of his numerous and rigorous scientific tests that show primary perception is a predictable form of ongoing bio-communication. His research has been replicated as far back as 1972 by Russian researcher V.N. Pushkin. Pushkin's experiments used people who were apparently hypnotically sophisticated and made use of hypnotic suggestions to evoke emotional imagery. Just as in Backster's original experiments, monitored plant cells showed a measurable response.

I interpret this to mean that cells have a mode of communication that is not exclusively reliant on a nervous system. Based on this and other evidence, we know that when both hypnotherapist and client are in just the right state of hypnotic rapport, the use of proper emotionalized imagery exerts a positive healing influence on the client's body at the cellular level.

Braud, also interested in the influence of thought upon biological structures at a distance, set up another fairly simple experiment with human cells. He put red blood cells in a container with a sodium solution. He used a hypotonic saline solution (too little sodium in the solution), which would normally cause the red blood cells to superhydrate and rupture. He wanted to see if a person could transfer their positive intention to the red blood cells and delay the bloating and rupturing that would normally occur in a hypotonic solution. Braud had people send thoughts and images telling the red blood cells to stay intact.

The experiment was a success. The act of mentally sending the positive intention was successful in protecting the red blood cells, allowing them to survive much longer than would normally be possible in a hypotonic saline solution. You can read more about research conducted by Braud and his colleagues in his book *Distant Mental Influence.*

This kind of research is beginning to explain how healing imagery and the thoughts we hold about our clients influence the results they achieve. Recently, Robert Sapien and I presented some of our methods at the annual International Conference on Science and Consciousness. We were among some of the preeminent scientists and authors in the field of consciousness research—people like Russell Targ, Cleve Backster, Christine Page, James O'Dea, Marilyn Schlitz, Dan Millman and Gregg Braden. During Gregg Braden's presentation, he made the point that if we can understand what sets up a miracle, the "technology" behind it, we can turn it into a skill. By combining research like that mentioned above and clinical hypnotherapy methods, we're definitely on our way.

Noetigenesis™ and the Noetigenic Field

Since there was not yet a term in the literature that accurately described this phenomenon of direct creation through mind activity, I developed one. The ancient Greek philosopher Anaxagorus believed that mind, or what we might call consciousness, influenced the creation of all things. His word for this was *nous.* Using this and the related Greek words *noetikos* and *noetic* and combining them with the word *genesis,* meaning creation, I've coined the term—Noetigenesis™ (pronounced no-EH-ti-JEN-eh-sis). Noetigenesis means direct creation through mind activity.

Your positive thoughts about your client accumulate to form your intention for them. And scientific research now shows that intention has a reliable effect at the cellular level, even when the object of your intention lacks a nervous system. This kind of intentional influence at a distance is what I call Noetigenics. The healing application of Noetigenics™ I refer to as Noetigenic Healing.™

Fundamental to understanding Noetigenic Healing is the concept of the Noetigenic Field. A field, in this case, refers to the sphere of influence of some force. With the Noetigenic Field, that force is consciousness itself. The Noetigenic Field is the, as yet unidentified, healing matrix that connects you with your client and makes Noetigenic Healing possible.

Noetigenics and the Noetigenic Field have been used intentionally or unintentionally in the ancient shamanic and Native American healing traditions for ages, as well by mesmerists and hypnotists throughout the eighteenth, nineteenth, and twentieth centuries. One twentieth century hypnotherapist who made intentional use of the Noetigenic Field is Emile Coué. He facilitated phenomenal results with a wide variety of people, including many so-called terminally ill patients. Part of what Coué did was to hold the thought-picture of his client's ideal healthy state vividly in his mind, thereby generating a Noetigenic Field of healing probability. Coué believed that if he held an image of the client as fully healed clearly enough in his own mind, that

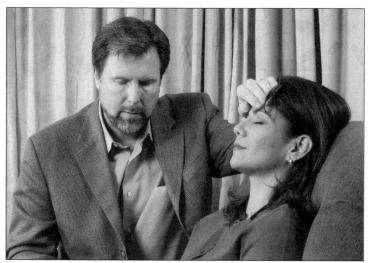
Generating a Noetigenic Field of healing probability

image would then exist in the mind of the client and act as healing imagery for them.

Coué also stressed that, in order for this method to succeed, the client had to truly desire their own healing. This is what I mean when I say that healing happens best when two or more gather to create a perfect thought-union. The singular purpose of the thought-union is to see the client as joyfully whole.

The first skill needed for Noetigenic Healing™ is the ability to develop a positive intention for every patient or client. When they are in hypnosis, you must vividly picture them free of pain and fully healed. Do this when guiding them through therapeutic suggestions and healing imagery. Imagine that you are speaking directly to the intelligence of the parts of the body affected by their temporary disease or injury. You see the cancer cells vanishing and being replaced by new healthy cells and tissue, and so on.

Other Noetigenic Healing™ skills will be presented in volume 2, *Medical Hypnotherapy*.

APPENDIX A

Two-Finger Eye Closure, Arm Drop, Trance Termination

Begin with the Two Finger Eye Closure induction.

> "Begin by finding a nice spot high on the ceiling to stare at… Now take in a nice, deep breath… Now open your eyes as wide as you can… Take another deep breath, keeping your eyes open wide… Now I'm going to close them with my finger and thumb."

Reach over and gently guide the client's eyes closed with one finger and thumb. Your forefinger and thumb come to rest on the client's cheekbones, with a slight pressure on the eyelids.

> "Now relax the eyelid muscles beneath my finger and thumb."

Pause 5 seconds.

> "Now as I pull away my hand, continue relaxing the eyelids fully and completely. In fact, I want you to relax those eyelids so much that they just won't work."

Pause 5 seconds.

> "When you feel that you have relaxed them to the point where they just won't work, nod your head."

Client nods.

> "Now go ahead and test them. Test them, and when you're satisfied that they just won't work, say 'satisfied' out loud."

Client says, "Satisfied."

> "Now send that relaxation that's around the eyes all the way down through your body, down to the very tips of your toes."

Now deepen with an Arm Drop.

> "In a moment I am going to lift your arm up and drop it like this."

Lift the client's arm up about six inches, gripping it either by the wrist or by the thumb, and then gently place it back down. Be conscious of anatomy.

> "When I do, just let your arm be loose, limp, and heavy. Let me have the full weight of your arm and let me do all the lifting. And when I drop the arm, just let it plop down. I will then say the words 'sleep deeply.' 'Sleep deeply' is your signal to double your relaxation. Alright, I'm going to pick up your arm now."

Now lift the client's arm just as you demonstrated. Notice whether or not they have responded to your suggestions to relax their arm and let you do all the lifting. If you notice that they are still tense or that they are helping you lift the arm, you can gently wiggle the arm while using patter to help them relax it completely. When the arm is completely relaxed, drop it and say:

"Sleep deep and double your relaxation."

DELIVER ACCELERATED HEALING AND PAIN CONTROL TECHNIQUES, THERAPEUTIC SUGGESTIONS, AND HEALING IMAGERY HERE.

When the session is finished, terminate the trance as follows:

"Alright, (person's name), in a moment I will count from one up to five. As I do, bring yourself out of hypnosis and bring with you all the peace and comfort you are now experiencing. When I say the number five, you will then open your eyes, stretch, and smile, and be fully alert.

One… Slowly, calmly, and gently bring yourself up and out of hypnosis. All the good, comfortable sensations stay with you as you come out of hypnosis.

Two… Each muscle in your body is loose, limp, and relaxed. You feel good. Your body continues to heal itself rapidly now. Each and every time you practice hypnosis, you respond more profoundly, going deeper into relaxation with every session.

Three… As you bring yourself up and out of hypnosis you feel wonderful in every way. You are emotionally calm and serene, physically at ease, and mentally clear and alert. You look forward to practicing hypnosis again.

Four… Preparing to open your eyes on the next number. In a moment, when you open your eyes, you are fully alert, noticing how good you feel.

Five… Eyes open now. Stretch, smile, and notice how good you feel."

APPENDIX B

Flashlight, Eye Closure, Arm Drop Trance Termination

Begin with the Flashlight induction.

> "Would you like me to show you an easy way to go into hypnosis so you can feel better?"

Position the penlight about twelve inches from the client's face and up about 45 degrees above their line of sight. Aim the beam at the tip of the client's nose.

> "Now look at the light and keep your eyes open while I count backwards from five down to one. When I reach the number one, just close your eyes and you will be in a pleasant state of hypnosis."

As you slowly count backwards (script follows), move the light down towards the client's face in an arc. Keep the beam of light pointed at the tip of the nose throughout the entire movement. By the time you reach the number one, your hand should at the level of the client's chin, with the beam angled up slightly toward the nose.

> "Five… Staring at the light takes you into hypnosis, and your eyes automatically become heavy and tired.
>
> Four… Looking at the light, your eyes begin to feel heavy and tired as if sleepy.

> Three... Your eyes are getting heavier and heavier. Blinking is hypnosis coming on.
>
> Two... It will feel so good to close your eyes, and relax.
>
> One... Just close your eyes down as you drift even deeper and deeper relaxed."

Move the light away and turn the beam off. The client is now in hypnosis and you can deepen with Eye Closure.

> "Now (person's name), put all of your attention on your eyelids. Relax your eyelid muscles completely. Relax the upper eyelids and the lower eyelids fully and completely. Relax the eyelids so much that they just won't work."

Pause for 5 seconds.

> "When you have relaxed them so much that you are sure that they just won't work, nod your head."

Client nods.

> "Now go ahead and test them. Test them, and find that they just won't work."

Give the client a few seconds to try to open their eyes unsuccessfully, then continue with the following.

> "Wonderful. Stop trying now and notice how good that feels. Now send that relaxation that you have in and around your eyes all throughout your body,

from the top of your head down to the tips of your toes."

Now deepen with an Arm Drop.

"In a moment I am going to lift your arm up and drop it like this."

Lift the client's arm up about six inches, gripping it either by the wrist or by the thumb, and then gently place it back down. Be conscious of anatomy.

"When I do, just let your arm be loose, limp, and heavy. Let me have the full weight of your arm and let me do all the lifting. And when I drop the arm, just let it plop down. I will then say the words 'sleep deeply.' 'Sleep deeply' is your signal to double your relaxation. Alright, I'm going to pick up your arm now."

Now lift the client's arm just as you demonstrated. Notice if they have responded to your suggestions to relax their arm and let you do all the lifting. If you notice that they are still tense or that they are helping you lift the arm, you can gently wiggle the arm while using patter to help them relax it completely. When the arm is completely relaxed, drop it and say:

"Sleep deeply and double your relaxation."

DELIVER ACCELERATED HEALING AND PAIN CONTROL TECHNIQUES, THERAPEUTIC SUGGESTIONS, AND HEALING IMAGERY HERE.

When the session is finished, terminate the trance.

"Alright, (person's name), in a moment I will count from one up to five. As I do, bring yourself out of hypnosis and bring with you all the peace and comfort you are now experiencing. When I say the number five, you will then open your eyes, stretch, and smile, and be fully alert.

One… Slowly, calmly, and gently bring yourself up and out of hypnosis. All the good, comfortable sensations stay with you as you come out of hypnosis.

Two… Each muscle in your body is loose, limp, and relaxed. You feel good. Your body continues to heal itself rapidly now. Each and every time you practice hypnosis, you respond more profoundly, going deeper into relaxation with every session.

Three… As you bring yourself up and out of hypnosis you feel wonderful in every way. You are emotionally calm and serene, physically at ease, and mentally clear and alert. You look forward to practicing hypnosis again.

Four… Preparing to open your eyes on the next number. In a moment, when you open your eyes, you are fully alert, noticing how good you feel.

Five… Eyes open now. Stretch, smile, and notice how good you feel."

APPENDIX C

Ideomotor/Pendulum, Arm Drop, Progressive Relaxation, Trance Termination

Begin with the Ideomotor induction.

> "I want to show you a hypnosis method that also teaches you how to direct the power of your subconscious mind. Shall we begin?"

When the client responds in the affirmative, give them the pendulum and have them hold it out in from of them between their index finger and thumb.

> "Now I want you to stare directly at the pendulum and hold it as steady as possible. As you look at the pendulum, vividly imagine it swinging side to side just like a clock pendulum swings side to side. (Person's name), picture the pendulum swinging side to side. Just use the power of your mind to move the pendulum. Want it to happen… See it happening… Then it happens…"

Pause for about 5 seconds to give them time before continuing.

> "That's it, just imagine the pendulum swinging side to side, and it swings side to side. Just watch what happens to the pendulum."

Watch the pendulum yourself, and be encouraging as the movement begins. Some people will so successfully picture the pendulum swinging that the movement begins in only 5 to 10 seconds. Others may take 15 to 20 seconds to get some movement.

After the client has the pendulum swinging side to side, simply by visualizing it, have them change the direction of the movement so that the pendulum swings either in a circle or toward and away from them.

> **"Good, you are doing very well. Now I want you to change the movement of the pendulum so that it swings either in a circle or toward and away from you. Once you've chosen the new movement, just picture and vividly imagine the pendulum swinging in that new direction. Just use the power of your mind to move the pendulum. Want it to happen... See it happening... Then it happens."**

Occasionally the client will need a little more guidance in order to get their mind focused on the correct imagery to bring about the desired movement in the pendulum. You can help by repeating and embellishing the instructions for them.

After the client has the pendulum swinging in the new direction, you can be assured they have established contact with their subconscious and it has become responsive to their instruction. They are putting themselves into hypnosis. Now it's time to deepen the experience. Speak in a calm, melodious voice as you give the following instructions.

> **"Now as you watch the pendulum, let your arm and eyes begin to get heavy and tired feeling...**

> Notice what happens as your arm gets even heavier now. Your eyes are on the pendulum, and your arm is getting so heavy, that it begins to slowly pull down, towards your lap…
>
> That's right, and as soon as the pendulum touches your lap, your eyes close and you'll be in a pleasant state of hypnosis…
>
> Your arm is getting heavier and heavier, pulling down… down… down to your lap. You may notice that even your eyes are feeling heavy… heavy… heavy and tired…
>
> As soon as the pendulum touches your lap, your eyes close and you are in that pleasant state of hypnosis…"

The pendulum touches their lap and their eyes close. This is an excellent time to begin conditioning the client to use self-hypnosis. Reach over, gently touch client's forehead as you say the following.

> "Sleep now. When I say, 'sleep now' I'm not referring the kind of sleep you sleep at night. I'm referring to this pleasant hypnotic state where you have released stress and tension and you are relaxed. Whenever you want to go into hypnosis, you can use your pendulum and when it touches your lap, just say 'sleep now' and you easily and immediately go into a pleasant hypnotic state. Not because I say so, but because it's the nature and ability of your subconscious mind to do so."

Now deepen with an Arm Drop.

> "In a moment I am going to lift your arm up and drop it like this."

Lift the client's arm up about six inches, gripping it either by the wrist or by the thumb, and then gently place it back down. Be conscious of anatomy.

> "When I do, just let your arm be loose, limp, and heavy. Let me have the full weight of your arm and let me do all the lifting. And when I drop the arm, just let it plop down. I will then say the words 'sleep deeply.' 'Sleep deeply' is your signal to double your relaxation. Alright, I'm going to pick up your arm now."

Now lift the client's arm just as you demonstrated. Notice whether or not they have responded to your suggestions to relax their arm and let you do all the lifting. If you notice that they are still tense or that they are helping you lift the arm, you can gently wiggle the arm while using patter to help them relax it completely. When the arm is completely relaxed, drop it and say:

> "Sleep deeply and double your relaxation."

Now deepen with a Progressive Relaxation.

> "Now to go even deeper relaxed and become even more responsive to positive healing ideas, begin to relax all the muscles in your scalp. You are safe, and you begin to feel a great wave of peace flow over you. Imagine a warm, relaxing feeling moving into your

neck. Think about all the neck muscles becoming loose and limp."

Pause a few seconds to allow the client to think about and experience the relaxation.

> "Now slowly and gently move the warm relaxation into your shoulders and down into your arms. Just use the power of your imagination. Just imagine the muscles turning loose and limp and relaxing more and more. Your shoulders, arms, and hands are becoming pleasantly warm and relaxed."

Pause a few seconds.

> "Move the comfortable relaxing sensation down your back now. Imagine, sense, and feel that you are sending the warm relaxing energy into all the muscles of your back. Picture all the back muscles loosening and relaxing now."

Pause a few seconds.

> "You are becoming more deeply relaxed and at peace now. Send the warm, relaxing sensation down into your hips and legs. Slowly, easily, and gently, imagine the relaxing sensation melting away any tension as the warm, relaxing, comfortable feeling moves down, down, down into your legs."

Pause a few seconds.

> "Send the relaxing sensation down past your ankles now and into your feet. Your feet and toes are becoming

warm and relaxed and comfortable now, and your subconscious mind is open and will act upon positive healing ideas. Just being in this hypnotic relaxation is healing for you, (person's name). Enjoy this pleasant time as your body restores itself to perfect health."

DELIVER ACCELERATED HEALING AND PAIN CONTROL TECHNIQUES, THERAPEUTIC SUGGESTIONS, AND HEALING IMAGERY HERE.

When the session is finished, terminate the trance.

"Alright, (person's name), in a moment I will count from one up to five. As I do, bring yourself out of hypnosis and bring with you all the peace and comfort you are now experiencing. When I say the number five, you will then open your eyes, stretch, and smile, and be fully alert.

One… Slowly, calmly, and gently bring yourself up and out of hypnosis. All the good, comfortable sensations stay with you as you come out of hypnosis.

Two… Each muscle in your body is loose, limp, and relaxed. You feel good. Your body continues to heal itself rapidly now. Each and every time you practice hypnosis, you respond more profoundly, going deeper into relaxation with every session.

Three… As you bring yourself up and out of hypnosis you feel wonderful in every way. You are emotionally calm and serene, physically at ease, and mentally clear and alert. You look forward to practicing hypnosis again.

Four… Preparing to open your eyes on the next number. In a moment, when you open your eyes, you are fully alert, noticing how good you feel.

Five… Eyes open now. Stretch, smile, and notice how good you feel."

APPENDIX D

Two-Finger Eye Closure, Repeated Eye Closure, Arm Drop, Disappearing Numbers Trance Termination

Begin with the Two Finger Eye Closure induction.

> "Begin by finding a spot high on the ceiling to stare at… Now take in a nice, deep breath… Now open your eyes as wide as you can… Take another deep breath, keeping your eyes open wide… Now I'm going to close your eyes with my finger and thumb."

Reach over and gently guide the client's eyes closed with one finger and thumb. Your forefinger and thumb come to rest on the client's cheekbones, with a slight bit of pressure on the eyelids.

> "Now relax the eyelid muscles beneath my finger and thumb."

Pause 5 seconds.

> "Now as I pull away my hand, continue relaxing the eyelids fully and completely. In fact, I want you to relax those eyelids so much that they just won't work."

Pause 5 seconds.

> "When you feel that you have relaxed them to the point where they just won't work, nod your head."

Client nods.

> "Now go ahead and test them. Test them, and when you're satisfied that they just won't work, say 'satisfied' out loud."

Client says, "Satisfied."

> "Now send that relaxation that's around the eyes all the way down through your body, down to the very tips of your toes."

Now deepen with Repeated Eye Closure.

> "In a moment I'll ask you to open and close your eyes. Each time I have you open and close your eyes, your physical relaxation will double. Just want that to happen and it will happen. Alright, open your eyes… Now close your eyes and let your physical relaxation double. Just let go and feel your body relaxing. Let that feeling of relaxation go all throughout your body, (person's name)."

Pause a few seconds to allow the client to deepen their relaxation.

> "In a moment I'll ask you to open and close your eyes again. And again, when you close your eyes, double this physical relaxation. Okay, open your

eyes... Now close your eyes. Close them and you're going way down... deeper... deeper relaxed. Send the relaxation all throughout your body now."

Pause a few seconds to allow the client to deepen their relaxation.

"Good. And now let's do that one more time. Go ahead and open your eyes... And just let them close down and double your physical relaxation again. Really letting go. Going down... down... deeper relaxed. Send that feeling throughout your whole body now."

Now deepen with an Arm Drop.

"In a moment I am going to lift your arm up and drop it like this."

Lift the client's arm up about six inches, gripping it either by the wrist or by the thumb, and then gently place it back down. Be conscious of anatomy.

"When I do, just let your arm be loose, limp, and heavy. Let me have the full weight of your arm and let me do all the lifting. And when I drop the arm, just let it plop down. I will then say the words 'sleep deeply.' 'Sleep deeply' is your signal to double your relaxation. Alright, I'm going to pick up your arm now."

Now lift the client's arm just as you demonstrated. Notice whether or not they have responded to your suggestions to relax their arm and let you do all the lifting. If you notice that they are still tense or that they are helping you lift the arm, you can gently wiggle the arm while using patter to help them relax it completely. When the arm is completely relaxed, drop it and say:

> "Sleep deeply and double your relaxation."

Now deepen with Disappearing Numbers.

> "Now that you are physically relaxed, I want to show you how to mentally relax. You see, (person's name), when you relax your mind, you can do anything. We want your mind to be just as relaxed as your body. So, when I tell you to, I want you to start counting backward from 100 out loud. For each number, starting at 100, first say the number out loud. Then I want you to double your mental relaxation as you make the number disappear completely from your mind. You'll say the number, then relax it out, sending it out of your mind. Then, when that number is gone, say, 'Faded away.' Then say the next number, and relax it out of your mind, and so on. By the time you reach 97, you will be so mentally relaxed that all numbers will have completely disappeared from your mind temporarily.
>
> Alright, begin by saying, '100,' then double your relaxation and send it out of your mind. When it's completely gone from your mind, say, 'Faded away.'"

Client says, "100."

> "Make it disappear as you double your mental relaxation. When it's completely gone from your mind, say, 'Faded away.'"

D – Two-Finger Eye Closure with Disappearing Numbers

Client says, "Faded away."

"Now say the next number, and then make it disappear as you double your mental relaxation."

Client says, "99."

"Make it disappear as you double your mental relaxation. When it's completely gone from your mind, say, 'Faded away.'"

Client says, "Faded away."

"Good. Say the next number, and then make it disappear as you double your mental relaxation again."

Client says, "98."

"Now make it disappear as you double your mental relaxation. When it's completely gone from your mind, say, 'Faded away.'"

Client says, "Faded away."

"Good. All the numbers are fading right out of your mind now. Just continue counting and doubling your mental relaxation on each number until all the numbers are completely gone."

Client says, "97."

"Double your mental relaxation. When it's gone, just say, 'Faded away.'"

Client says, "Faded away."

"Numbers faded away completely now… When all the numbers are gone from your mind, just say, 'Gone.'"

Client says, "Gone."

"Now let your mind be filled with nothingness."

DELIVER ACCELERATED HEALING AND PAIN CONTROL TECHNIQUES, THERAPEUTIC SUGGESTIONS, AND HEALING IMAGERY HERE.

When the session is finished, terminate the trance.

"Alright, (person's name), in a moment I will count from one up to five. As I do, bring yourself out of hypnosis and bring with you all the peace and comfort you are now experiencing. When I say the number five, you will then open your eyes, stretch, and smile, and be fully alert.

One… Slowly, calmly, and gently bring yourself up and out of hypnosis. All the good, comfortable sensations stay with you as you come out of hypnosis.

Two… Each muscle in your body is loose, limp, and relaxed. You feel good. Your body continues to heal itself rapidly now. Each and every time you practice hypnosis, you respond more profoundly, going deeper into relaxation with every session.

Three… As you bring yourself up and out of hypnosis you feel wonderful in every way. You are emotionally calm and serene, physically at ease, and mentally clear and alert. You look forward to practicing hypnosis again.

Four… Preparing to open your eyes on the next number. In a moment, when you open your eyes, you are fully alert, noticing how good you feel.

Five… Eyes open now. Stretch, smile, and notice how good you feel."

APPENDIX E

Hand Press, Head Roll, Arm Drop, Eye Catalepsy, Progressive Relaxation, Trance Termination

Begin with the Hand Press induction.

> "Would you like to learn a way to go into hypnosis instantly?"

Client responds in the affirmative. Holding your hand out, palm up, say the following with a firm, strong voice.

> "Okay, put your hand on mine. Now start pushing down on my hand. I want you to press firmly."

Point to your eye with your free hand as you say the following.

> "Now I want you to look directly into my eye."

While client is looking into your eye, continue.

> "Look into my eye and go into hypnosis. As you look into my eye, your eyes start to get heavy and tired. Each time they blink, that's hypnosis coming on. Eyes are getting heavy, droopy, and drowsy."

Move your non-pressing hand very slowly toward the client's face to non-verbally communicate that you want them to close their eyes and continue with the following:

> **"Now eyes closing... closing... closing... Eyes getting heavier, tired and closing now. Closing them."**

The moment the eyes close and stay closed for about one or two seconds, immediately strengthen your voice and deliver the sleep command as you simultaneously jerk your hand out from underneath the client's hand so that they lurch forward slightly. A slight loss of equilibrium helps to induce the trance.

> **"SLEEP!"**

Then gently push the client's head back to the recliner chair and rock their head side to side about an inch or two for deepening the trance. If the client is not sitting or lying such that they have a surface to support their head, you can also lean their head forward so that their forehead is cradled by your hand and rock it back and forth that way.

> **"Now, you are going deep into hypnosis. Neck muscles relaxing and letting go. Let me gently rock your head side to side while you go deeper and deeper. Your neck muscles are becoming loose and limp and relaxed now. When I use the word sleep, I am not referring to the kind of sleep you sleep at night. I am referring to this hypnotic state you are now experiencing."**

After slowly rocking the head side to side three or four times, move on to deepening with an Arm Drop.

> "In a moment I am going to lift your arm up and drop it like this."

Lift the client's arm up about six inches, gripping it either by the wrist or by the thumb, and then gently place it back down. Be conscious of anatomy.

> "When I do, just let your arm be loose, limp, and heavy. Let me have the full weight of your arm and let me do all the lifting. And when I drop the arm, just let it plop down. I will then say the words 'sleep deeply.' 'Sleep deeply' is your signal to double your relaxation. Alright, I'm going to pick up your arm now."

Now lift the client's arm just as you demonstrated. Notice whether or not they have responded to your suggestions to relax their arm and let you do all the lifting. If you notice that they are still tense or that they are helping you lift the arm, you can gently wiggle the arm while using patter to help them relax it completely. When the arm is completely relaxed, drop it and say:

> "Sleep deeply and double your relaxation."

Now deepen with an Eye Catalepsy.

> "In a moment I am going to count backwards from five down to one and you are going to experience your highly responsive subconscious mind doing it's perfect work for you. On or before the number one, your eyelids are locked down tight. Any attempt to open them causes them to lock down tighter."

Place your finger on the bridge of their nose, just between the eyebrows.

> "Five… Eyelids locking down tight.
>
> Four… Eyelids sealing shut, as if glued.
>
> Three… Eyelids pressing down and sealing shut.
>
> Two… Any attempt to open your eyes causes them to lock down tighter."

Pull away your hand.

> "One… Try to open your eyes and find them locking down tight."

Pause a few seconds while the client attempts to open their eyes, then continue.

> "Alright, stop trying and go three times deeper into hypnosis."

Now deepen with a Progressive Relaxation.

> "Now to go even deeper relaxed and become even more responsive to positive healing ideas, begin to relax all the muscles in your scalp. You are safe, and you begin to feel a great wave of peace flow over you. Imagine a warm, relaxing feeling moving into your neck. Think about all the neck muscles becoming loose and limp."

Pause a few seconds to allow the client to think about and experience the relaxation.

"Now slowly and gently move the warm relaxation into your shoulders and down into your arms. Just use the power of your imagination. Just imagine the muscles turning loose and limp and relaxing more and more. Your shoulders, arms, and hands are becoming pleasantly warm and relaxed."

Pause a few seconds.

"Move the comfortable relaxing sensation down your back now. Imagine, sense, and feel that you are sending the warm relaxing energy into all the muscles of your back. Picture all the back muscles loosening and relaxing now."

Pause a few seconds.

"You are becoming more deeply relaxed and at peace now. Send the warm, relaxing sensation down into your hips and legs. Slowly, easily, and gently, imagine the relaxing sensation melting away any tension as the warm, relaxing, comfortable feeling moves down, down, down into your legs."

Pause a few seconds.

"Send the relaxing sensation down past your ankles now and into your feet. Your feet and toes are becoming warm and relaxed and comfortable now, and your subconscious mind is open and will act upon positive healing ideas. Just being in this hypnotic relaxation is healing for you, (person's name). Enjoy this pleasant time as your body restores itself to perfect health."

DELIVER ACCELERATED HEALING AND PAIN CONTROL TECHNIQUES, THERAPEUTIC SUGGESTIONS, AND HEALING IMAGERY HERE.

When the session is finished, terminate the trance.

> "Alright, (person's name), in a moment I will count from one up to five. As I do, bring yourself out of hypnosis and bring with you all the peace and comfort you are now experiencing. When I say the number five, you will then open your eyes, stretch, and smile, and be fully alert.
>
> One… Slowly, calmly, and gently bring yourself up and out of hypnosis. All the good, comfortable sensations stay with you as you come out of hypnosis.
>
> Two… Each muscle in your body is loose, limp, and relaxed. You feel good. Your body continues to heal itself rapidly now. Each and every time you practice hypnosis, you respond more profoundly, going deeper into relaxation with every session.
>
> Three… As you bring yourself up and out of hypnosis you feel wonderful in every way. You are emotionally calm and serene, physically at ease, and mentally clear and alert. You look forward to practicing hypnosis again.
>
> Four… Preparing to open your eyes on the next number. In a moment, when you open your eyes, you are fully alert, noticing how good you feel.
>
> Five… Eyes open now. Stretch, smile, and notice how good you feel."

APPENDIX F

Sequential Imagery, Trance Termination

Begin with the Sequential Imagery induction.

"Please take a good, long, deep breath and close your eyes. Now make yourself comfortable and prepare for a very enjoyable journey. Imagine you are outside. It's a bright, sunny day, and there is a gentle breeze. Imagine you are standing at the top of a set of ten steps that lead down to a warm and inviting beach. The stairway is very sturdy because it is set in the earth. Put a handrail on both sides of the stairway. Look at the steps. There are ten steps. There are ten steps and they are numbered. The top step has the number ten on it, the next step has a nine on it, and so on all the way down to the last step, which has the number one on it. The last step, which is at the bottom, is on the beach.

In a moment I will begin counting backwards. As I do, vividly imagine that you are slowly walking down the steps. Go down one step with each number I speak. With each step you will go deeper and deeper into hypnotic relaxation. On the number one you will be on the last step and eager to step off into the warm sand.

Alright. Number ten… Imagine, sense, and feel yourself step down, going down deeper into hypnosis.

Number nine… Step down. Going down deeper, deeper, and deeper relaxed with each step you imagine yourself taking. Imagine the warm breeze is becoming real for you. You imagine the smell of the salt air.

Number eight… See the number eight written on the step and step down, going deeper and deeper relaxed.

Number seven… Step down. Going down deeper, deeper, and deeper relaxed with each step you imagine yourself taking. The big blue sky has a few clouds in it and you can hear the call of seagulls now that you are getting closer to the bottom of the stairs.

Number six… Imagine, sense, and feel that you are stepping down onto the sixth step, and you are going deeper and deeper relaxed.

Five… Step down. Put yourself halfway down the steps. You are halfway to the warm sandy beach at the bottom of the stairs."

Start slowing your speech pattern slightly now.

"Four… Step down to the fourth step. And go down deeper, deeper, and deeper relaxed with each step you imagine yourself taking.

Number three… You are almost there on the beach.

Two… Down, down, down, deeper, deeper, deeper.

> One... Step down onto the last step. In a moment you will step down onto the beach and go deeper into hypnosis. You're relaxing deeply and that feels good. Okay, imagine you are barefoot now and then step off into the warm sand.
>
> As you step into the sand you sink down about an inch into the soft, warm granules of sand. Put a lounge chair with a bright umbrella over it a few feet in front of you. Walk over to the lounge chair and get in it. The shade produced by the umbrella makes this place just the right temperature for you. Out in the distance you see the gentle ocean waves lapping back and forth on the sand. Here in this place of perfect serenity your subconscious mind is open and receptive to the beneficial ideas we spoke about before hypnosis."

DELIVER ACCELERATED HEALING AND PAIN CONTROL TECHNIQUES, THERAPEUTIC SUGGESTIONS, AND HEALING IMAGERY HERE.

When the session is finished, terminate the trance.

> "Alright, (person's name), in a moment I will count from one up to five. As I do, bring yourself out of hypnosis and bring with you all the peace and comfort you are now experiencing. When I say the number five, you will then open your eyes, stretch, and smile, and be fully alert.
>
> One... Slowly, calmly, and gently bring yourself up and out of hypnosis. All the good, comfortable sensations stay with you as you come out of hypnosis.

Two… Each muscle in your body is loose, limp, and relaxed. You feel good. Your body continues to heal itself rapidly now. Each and every time you practice hypnosis, you respond more profoundly, going deeper into relaxation with every session.

Three… As you bring yourself up and out of hypnosis you feel wonderful in every way. You are emotionally calm and serene, physically at ease, and mentally clear and alert. You look forward to practicing hypnosis again.

Four… Preparing to open your eyes on the next number. In a moment, when you open your eyes, you are fully alert, noticing how good you feel.

Five… Eyes open now. Stretch, smile, and notice how good you feel."

APPENDIX G

Elman's Magic Spot (Pediatric) Sapien/Simmerman Modified Version

Say to your patient:

"I'm going to give you a Magic Spot so that you can get some medicine without feeling anything, maybe some pressure like this? Would you like it on this arm, or that arm?" (appropriate body area for procedure)

"You are going to be really happy because the Magic Spot is amazing... Okay, let's play a game and I'll show you how to have a Magic Spot. I want you to open your eyes really wide..."

"Good, now just close them... All you have to do (patient's name) is pretend that you can't open your eyes... You and I know that if you wanted to, you could open them... But right now, I want you to pretend really hard that you can't open your eyes, and keep on pretending you can't open your eyes—so much that when you try to open your eyes, they just won't open..."

"Now let me see you try to open them while you're pretending... That's right..."

"Now stay like that, and keep on pretending that you can't open your eyes, and the most amazing thing is

> going to happen. You're going to have a Magic Spot where special cold alcohol is rubbed on your arm (body area of procedure). Once you have your Magic Spot, the nurse (medical personnel) can give you the medicine and it just won't bother you. You'll know that the nurse (medical personnel) is working there, and it's okay."

While medical personnel applies antiseptic continue by saying:

> "Okay, now the nurse (medical personnel) is painting on your Magic Spot. That's right, you keep on pretending that your eyes just won't open and you have a Magic Spot."

(Now medical personnel can proceed. Medical Hypnotist is to remember the Patter rule. (See page 73.) When you want to end the hypnosis proceed as follows)

> "Okay, I'm going to count to three and that's when you'll open your eyes and feel so much better... One... two... three..."

Bibliography and Suggested Reading

Anderson, Robert A. *The Scientific Basis for Wholistic Medicine.* East Wenatchee: American Health Press. 2004.

Backster, Cleve. *Primary Perception.* Anza: White Rose Millennium Press. 2002.

Baggaley, Ann, and Sara Freeman. *Human Body, An Illustrated Guide To Every Part Of The Human Body And How It Works.* London: Dorling Kindersley Limited. 2001.

Barber, Joseph. *Hypnosis and Suggestion in the Treatment of Pain.* New York: W.W. Norton & Company. 1996.

Boyce, Oren Douglas. *The Power of Indirect Suggestion, Hypnosis, Genetics, and Depression.* New York: Vantage. 1999.

Boyne, Gil. *How to Teach Self Hypnosis.* Glendale: Westwood Publishing Company, Inc. 1987.

Boyne, Gil. *Transforming Therapy.* Glendale: Westwood Publishing Company, Inc. 1989.

Boyne, Gil. *Instantaneous Inductions, Standing and Seated.* Glendale: Westwood Publishing Company, Inc. 1993.

Braden, Gregg. *The Isaiah Effect: Decoding the Lost Science of Prayer and Prophecy.* New York: Three Rivers Press. 2000.

Braud, William. *Distant Mental Influence.* Charlottesville: Hampton Roads Publishing Company, Inc. 2003.

Brooks, Harry C. *The Practice of Autosuggestion by the Method of Emile Coué.* Santa Fe: Sun Publishing Co. 1922.

Carpenter, Harry W. *The Genie Within, Your Subconscious Mind, How to Use It and How It Works.* San Diego: AnaphaseII Publishing. 2004.

Cialdini, Robert A. *Influence, Science And Practice.* Needham Heights: Allyn & Bacon. 2001.

Cheek, David B. and Ernest L. Rossi. *Mind-Body Therapy: Methods of Ideodynamic Healing in Hypnosis.* New York: W.W. Norton & Company. 1988.

Cohen, Harvey. *Adventures In Awareness.* Beverly Hills: AaaHa! Dynamic Press. 1992.

Coué, Emile. *Self Mastery through Conscious Autosuggestion.* Whitefish: Kessinger Publishing. 1922.

Custer, Dan. *The Miracle of Mind Power.* Glendale: Westwood Publishing Company, Inc. 1960.

Elman, Dave. *Hypnotherapy.* Glendale: Westwood Publishing Company, Inc. 1964.

Frost, Thomas. *Hypnosis in General Dental Practice.* London: Henry Kimton. 1959.

Hartland, John. *Medical and Dental Hypnosis, and its Clinical Applications.* 1971.

Holmes, Ernest. *The Science of Mind: A Philosophy, A Faith, A Way of Life.* New York: Penguin Putnam Inc. 1938.

Holmes, Ernest. *How to Use the Science of Mind.* Burbank: Science of Mind Publishing. 1948.

Jacobs, Donald Trent. *Patient Communication for First Responders and EMS Personnel.* Englewood Cliffs: Brady, A Prentice Hall Division. 1991.

Jampolsky, Gerald. *Love Is Letting Go of Fear.* Berkley: Celestial Arts. 1979.

Keyes, Ken. *The Hundredth Monkey.* Coos Bay: Vision Books. 1982.

Lewis, Allan. *Clearing Your Life Path through Kahuna Wisdom.* Las Vegas: Homana Publications. 1983.

Lipton, Bruce. *The Biology of Belief: Unleashing the Power of Consciousness, Matter and Miracles.* San Rafael: Mountain of Love Publishing. 2005.

McTaggart, Lynne. *The Field: The Quest for the Secret orce of the Universe.* New York: Harper Collins. 2002.

Murphy, Joseph. *The Power of Your Subconscious Mind.* New York: Bantam. 1963.

Powers, Melvin. *Hypnotism Revealed.* Los Angeles: Borden Publishing Company. 1969.

Prager, Judith Simon and Judith Acosta. *The Worst Is Over, What to Say When Every Moment Counts.* San Diego: Jodere Group, Inc. 2002.

Preston, Michael D. *Hypnosis: Medicine of the Mind. A Complete Manual on Hypnosis for the Beginner, Intermediate, and Advanced Practitioner.* Ulyssian Publications. 1998.

Ray, Sondra. *Loving Relationships.* Berkley: Celestial Arts. 1980.

Ray, Sondra. *Healing and Holiness.* Berkley: Celestial Arts. 2002.

Rossi, Ernest Lawrence. *The Psychobiology of Mind-Body Healing, New Concepts of Therapeutic Hypnosis.* New York: W.W. Norton & Company. 1986.

Shealy, C. Norman. *Miracles Do Happen: A Physician's Experience with Alternative Medicine.* London: Vega Books. 1995.

Scovel Shinn, Florence. *Your Word Is Your Wand.* Marina Del Ray: DeVorss & Co. 1928.

Siegel, Bernie. *Love, Medicine and Miracles.* New York: HarperCollins. 1986.

Sutphen, Dick. *Reinventing Yourself.* Malibu: Valley of the Sun Publishing. 1993.

Tebbitts, Charles. *Self Hypnosis and Other Mind Expanding Techniques.* Glendale: Westwood Publishing Company, Inc. 1987.

A Course in Miracles. Mill Valley: Foundation for Inner Peace. 1976.

Index

Active relaxation training, 196–200
Altered states, description and origins of, 17–19, 31–32
Analgesia versus anesthesia, 164–165
Arm catalepsy testing method, 91–93
Arm drop deepening method, 76–78, 211–225, 227–233, 235–240
Associated imagery, 119–120
Audio recordings, 190–192
Auditory imagery, 122–125
Autonomic nervous system, 21–25, 188, 201
Autosuggestion
  bypassing the critical faculty, 137
  duration of, 121–122
  saturating the mind with intentional autosuggestion, 189–196
Awareness, levels of, 26–29
Axiomatic signs of hypnosis, 47–48

Backster, Cleve, 205–206
Balloons and bucket exercise, 41–44
Beginner's mind, 53–54
Belief, 32
Boyne's Hand Press induction method, 65–68, 235–240
Change, client's desire for, 52–53
Competence-building strategy, 53–54
Concentration, 19
Conditioned response, killer stress as, 141–142
Consciousness, the science of, 205–207
Coué, Emile, 189, 208–209
Counting devices, 189–191, 194–195
Counting for trance termination, 71–72
Critical faculty, 17–19, 135–137

Danger, sympathetic nervous response to, 23–25
Daydreaming, 18
Deepening methods
  arm drop, 76–78, 211–225, 227–233, 235–240
  diaphragmatic breathing, 201
  disappearing numbers, 86–89, 227–233
  eye closure, 84–86, 227–233
  head roll, 78–79, 235–240
  progressive relaxation, 79–81, 219–225, 235–240
  reasons for, 75–76
  ten count method, 82–84
  warm light, 81–82
Dentistry, 120–122
Diaphragmatic breathing, 201
Dilution method of pain control, 155–161, 182–186
Diminution of pain, 147–154
Dissociation, 119–120, 179–186
Distraction, 34

Elman eye closure deepening
method, 84–85, 216–217
Elman's disappearing numbers,
86–89, 227–233
Emotion
associated and dissociated
imagery, 119–120
avoiding toxic thoughts,
187–188
bypassing the critical faculty,
136–137
creating scripts for healing, 99
fight-or-flight response,
23–25
characteristics of the hypnotic
state, 20–21
parasympathetic nervous
response, 25
subconscious use of language
of emotion, 28, 114
suffering as response to pain,
145–146
Ethics of self-hypnosis, 188–189
Excited imagination, 32–34
Expectancy, 32–34
beginner's mind, 53–54
fear-tension-pain cycle, 127–129
use of imagination to induce
positive expectancy, 38–39
Eye catalepsy, 89–91, 235–240
Eye closure methods, 54–56,
84–85, 211–214, 219–226,
227–233

Fear-tension-pain cycle, 127–129
Fight-or-flight response, 23–25
Finger clamp exercise, 39–41
Fixation, 34
Flashlight induction, 56–59, 73,
215–218
Forgiveness as healing agent,
144–145

Generalized Couism, 190
Glove anesthesia, 163–177

Hand press induction method,
65–68, 235–240
Head roll, 78–79, 235–240
Heightened responsiveness to
instruction, 20–21
High-self, 28
Homeostasis, 25
Huna tradition, 28
Hyperacuity of the senses, 49
Hypnosis defined, 17–19
Hypnotic state
axiomatic signs of, 47–48
characteristics of the hypnotic
state, 20–21
formula for hypnotic
induction, 32–36
terminating the trance, 71–72
See also Deepening methods;
Inducing hypnotic states;
Testing methods

Ideomotor movement, 59–64,
219–225
Imagery
associated versus dissociated,
119–120
creating healing imagery,
115–119
dilution method of pain
control, 155–161,
182–186
dream imagery, 27
influencing others' physiology
through, 205–209
sequential imagery as induction,
68–71, 241–244
speaking subconscious, 112
stating goals in positive terms,
111

use of the Noetigenic Field, 208–209
visual, auditory, and kinesthetic, 122–125
Imagination
  balloons and bucket exercise, 41–44
  finger clamp exercise, 39–41
  lemon exercise, 37–39
Immune system health, 187–201
Implied causative, 113
Inducing hypnotic states, 32–35
  correct use of patter, 73
  flashlight induction, 56–59, 73, 215–218
  hand press induction method, 65–68, 235–240
  ideomotor movement, 59–64, 219–225
  initial conditions, 51–53
  myth of the special induction, 49
  pendulum movement, 59–64, 219–225
  repeated eye closure, 85–86, 227–233
  sequential imagery, 68–71, 241–244
  terminating the trance, 71–72
  Two Finger Eye Closure technique, 54–56, 211–214, 227–233
Intuitive knowing, 29
"It" misconception, 45–47

Killer stress, 138–142
Kinesthetic imagery, 122–125

Language
  of emotion, 28
  hypnotic induction process, 33–35
  organ language, 138
  scripts to accelerate healing, 95–106
  speaking to the subconscious, 111–115
  using patter during induction, 73
Law of Impressed Thought, 107–108
Lemon exercise, 37–39, 107
Light, use of, 56–59, 73, 81–82, 215–218
Loved ones, illness and pain as connection with, 142–143

Mala, 189
Memory, 27
Mental relaxation, 86–89
Mind, 25–26
Misconceptions about hypnosis, 36, 45–46, 49
Motor movement as induction, 59–64
Myths. See Misconceptions about hypnosis

Negative payoff, 102–104
Nervous system. See Autonomic nervous system; Parasympathetic nervous system; Sympathetic nervous system
New age guilt, 102–103
Nocebo, 130–134
Noetigenesis, 207–209
Noetigenic Field, 208–209
Numeric sequences, use in induction, 68

Organ language, 138

Pain control and erasure
  amelioration by dissociation, 179–186

analgesia versus anesthesia, 164–165
dilution method, 155–161, 182–186
disappearing numbers, 86–89, 227–233
eliminating suffering, 145–146
fear-tension-pain cycle, 127–129
pain reduction by diminution, 147–149
placebo power, 129–130
use of autosuggestion, 120–121
using the mind's master controls, 149–154
Parasympathetic nervous system, 22(fig.), 23, 25, 47–48, 201
Patter, use of, 73
Pendulum movement as induction, 59–64, 219–225
Perception, power of, 21–23
Placebo power, 109, 129–134
Primary perception, 206
Progressive relaxation, 79–81, 219–225, 235–240

Realization, deepening through, 76
Refocused attention, 33–35
Relaxation
  characterizing the hypnotic state, 21, 48
  fear-tension-pain cycle, 127–129
  hypnotic induction process, 34
  supporting immune system health, 196–200
  See also Deepening methods; Inducing hypnotic states
Repeated eye closure deepening method, 85–86, 227–233
Repetition, 34, 136–137

Respiration as sign of hypnotic state, 49
Responsiveness to hypnosis, 31–49
  balloons and bucket exercise, 41–44
  debriefing responsiveness exercises, 45–47
  finger clamp exercise, 39–41
  lemon exercise, 37–38
  placebo power, 109
  refocusing attention, 33
  swing sway exercise, 44–45
Ritual, 34

Secondary gain, 102–104
Selective thinking, 17–19
Self-empowerment, 46, 59–64, 219–225
Self-esteem, 104–105, 139–141
Self-hypnosis, 64
  bypassing the critical faculty, 137
  ethics of, 188–189
  saturating the mind with intentional autosuggestion, 189–196
  script for teaching, 192–196
  scripting to facilitate, 105
Sensory imagery, 118–119, 155–161, 182–186
Sequential imagery, 68–71, 241–244
Shamanism, 31–32, 208–209
Signs of hypnosis, 49
Simmerman Model of the Triune Mind, 25–26
Speaking subconscious, 107–125
Startle command, 65–68
Stem sentence completion process, 98
Stress, 23–25, 138–142

Subconscious mind
  bypassing the critical faculty, 135–137
  dispelling the "it" misconception, 47
  excited imagination, 32–33
  lemon exercise using the imagination, 37–39
  memories of numbness, 163–164
  power of perception on the autonomic nervous system, 22–23, 22(fig.)
  subconscious level of awareness, 27–28
  using glove anesthesia, 167–168
Suffering meme, 143–144
Suggestion, 34, 37–39, 111
Superconscious level of awareness, 28–29
Survival mind, 23–25
Swing sway exercise, 44–45
Sympathetic nervous system, 22(fig.), 23–25

Tangled hierarchy, 21–23
Ten count for deepening, 82–84
Tension: fear-tension-pain cycle, 127–129
Testing methods
  arm catalepsy, 91–93
  eye catalepsy, 89–91, 235–240
  reasons for, 75–76
Therapeutic suggestions, 20
Time distortion, 49
Timing, importance of, 113–114
Touch, use of, 64–68, 235–240
Toxic thoughts, 187–188
Trance termination, 49, 71–72
Triune Mind, Simmerman Model of the, 25–26

Two finger eye closure method, 54–56, 211–214, 227–233
Universal Intelligence, 28
Vagus nerve stimulation, 201
Visual fixation, 56–59
Visual imagery, 122–125
Visualization. See Imagery
Warm light deepening method, 81–82

Hypnotherapy Academy of America

I look forward to hearing about the miracles you help to create using the methods I have shared with you in this book. If you are inspired to learn more about training in clinical hypnotherapy, see the Hypnotherapy Academy of America website at www.HypnotherapyAcademy.com where you will also find a schedule of classes.

Or to order copies of
Medical Hypnotherapy, volume 1
and a course catalog:

Call toll free 877-983-1515
For international calls 505-983-1515
Or visit our website: www.HypnotherapyAcademy.com

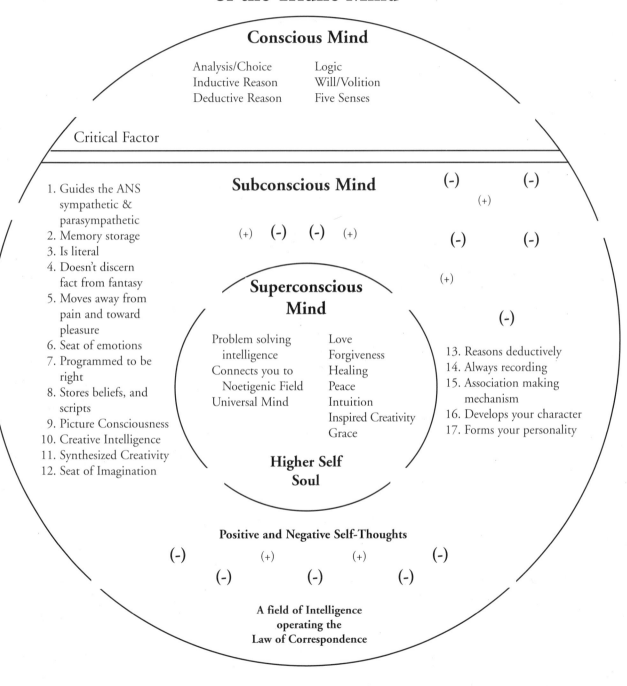